NATURAL PET PRODUCTIONS

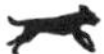

TAYLOR & BECKER

DR. BECKER'S REAL FOOD FOR HEALTHY DOGS & CATS

SIMPLE HOMEMADE FOOD

BETH TAYLOR & KAREN SHAW BECKER, DVM

For all the animals who share our lives, and especially for Gemini and Tessa, the dogs who showed us that real food can save lives.

Thanks to all the animals and people who keep us learning.

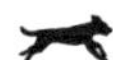

Disclaimer: The information in this book does not take the place of medical advice or veterinary care.

ISBN: 0982533101

Printed in the United States of America
Second Edition, First Printing: 2009

www.naturalpetproductions.com

photographs by Whitney Rupp, www.whitneyrupp.com
book design by Rosie Harper

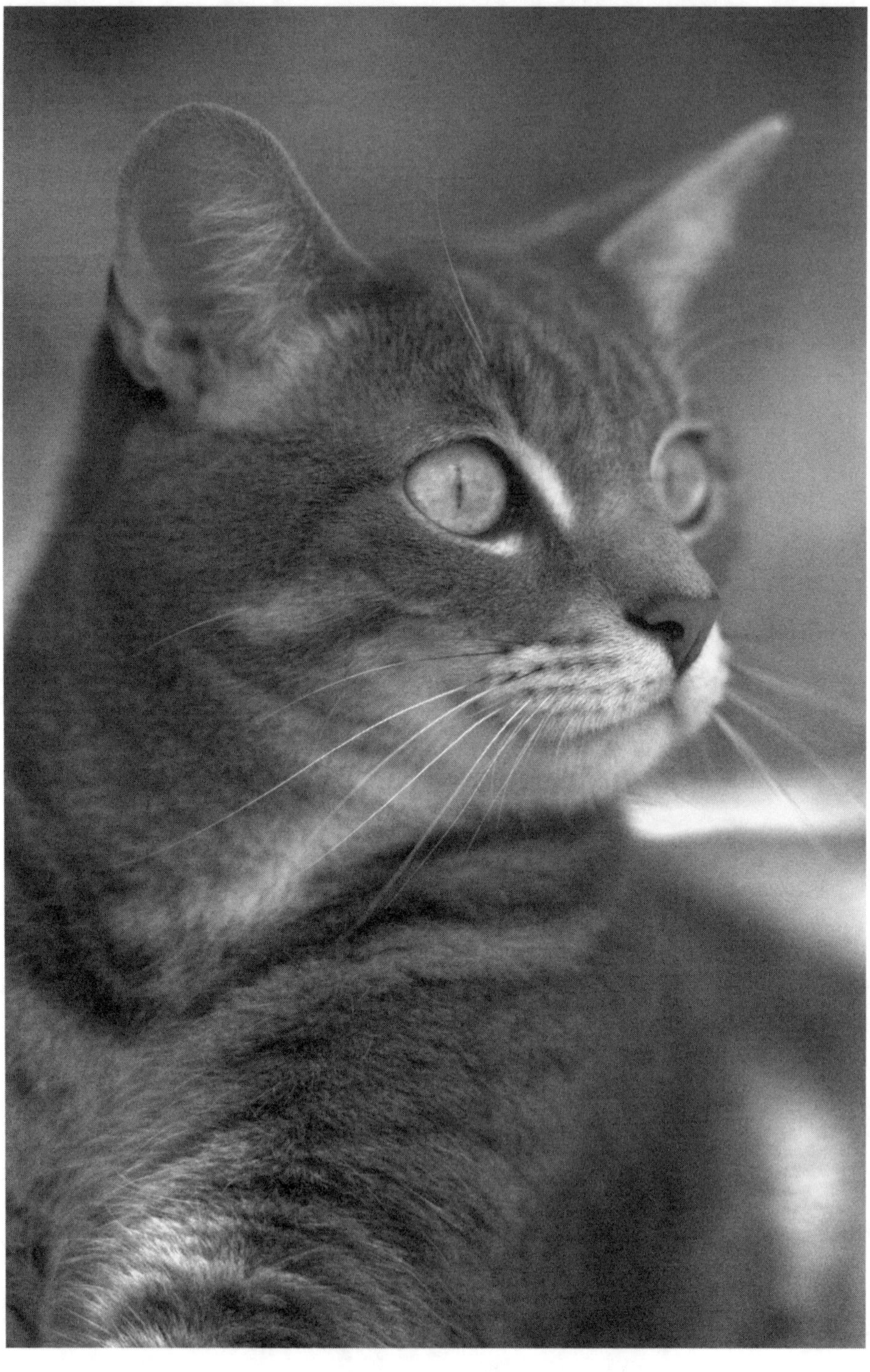

TABLE OF CONTENTS

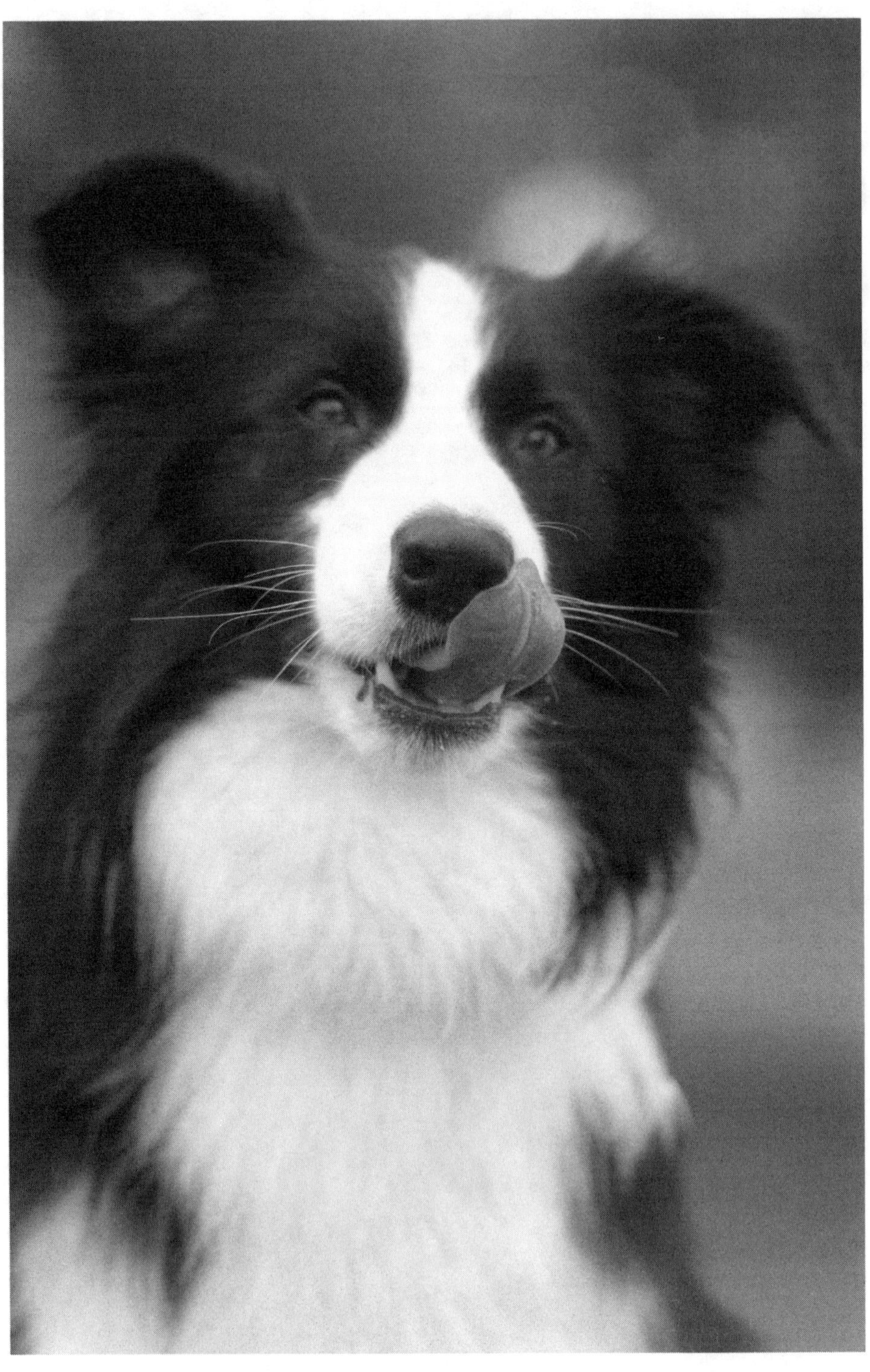

INTRODUCTION

We share our lives with animals because they're great companions. We want the same long and healthy lives for them that we want for ourselves. Good food, well-balanced relationships, clean air and water, plenty of exercise — these are all components of a healthy life.

We're told that humans need whole, minimally-processed foods, that we should vary our diets and eat fresh food. We often get different advice for our animals.

"Experts" say never to change your animal's diet. Never feed him people food. "Feed your dog complete food in a bag." Most of us accepted this concept for many years — though we would look for another doctor if we got this advice from our pediatricians.

We need convenience in our busy lives. We want food fast, for our animals and for ourselves. Dry food is the easy answer, the answer most of us accepted with little thought about the big picture of health. However, we are beginning to understand that there is no substitute for eating real food ourselves. The same is true for our animals. Many of the chronic and acute diseases suffered by humans and animals are directly related to diet.

The truth is, food is just food. There's no "dog food," "people food," "cat food," "bird food" — it's all just food, with the balance and ingredients differing depending on species. A fresh food diet is best for all living beings. A fresh, species-appropriate diet provides support for the body to maintain a vibrant state of being for many years. If your dog or cat is already bursting with health, you may not see a big difference when you switch to fresh food. If she has chronic health problems, you are likely to see those improve. You may notice that some of the small problems you thought were "just age" have diminished. Our advice: feed a fresh food diet. It's the most important component to promote a long and healthy life for your animals. And yourself. You might see such radical changes that you'll be inspired to overhaul your own diet!

Why would you want to make food yourself if you can buy good products? Making food for your pet is no small undertaking. Our culture is geared toward speed and convenience. The time it takes to prepare food can be considerable, but there are excellent reasons to make food for your pets.

Reasons to make food for your pets

- You can save a lot of money. If you use whole chickens and obtain a grinder, you can make chicken and veggie food for a quarter of the retail price. Even using separate body parts, your cost can be half the retail price. For turkey and beef, if you shop seasonally and watch sales, savings are similar. If your animal needs exotic protein sources, the savings will not be as great, but you'll still pay less for your food.

- You control the quality of ingredients when you make your own food. Pet food companies assert that they use top quality ingredients and claims of "organic" and "human-edible" may be true — or not. When you see cantaloupe on a label, does this mean a lovely, ripe piece of cantaloupe, or does it mean rinds left from the preparation of pre-cut fresh grocery store products, or whole cantaloupe with rinds? Cantaloupe rinds can harbor molds, fungicides and pesticides. For the manufacturer, these options represent lower production costs. For you, it's not such a good deal. Fat is another concern. When you make your own food, you know how much fat is really in there. Labels give the percentage of fat as a minimum. It could be more, and there is often variation between batches. These are just two examples of many different concerns.

- Food that's fresh tastes better and is more nutritious. Food you make is always fresher than food you buy. Several of our dogs, who leave commercial turkey food sitting in the bowl, became fans when we started to make it ourselves. Why? Was that commercial food "bad"? We don't think so. It just got a little old. It's still nutritionally balanced and ok to eat (though there is some nutrient loss in storage), but it doesn't taste as good. The long-term storage of commercial food affects nutrients enough that it's worth making your own food if you can find a way to fit it into your life.

You may be enthusiastic about preparing a fresh food diet for your pet. Or, you may be wondering how you're going to manage it. You might be convinced of the importance, but still worried about getting it "right." This book provides a sound framework. There are other ways to provide a fresh food diet. As you become more experienced and knowledgeable you may want to add variations. If you keep to the basic principles presented here, you'll do well.

These recipes have been analyzed and compared to the standards of both AAFCO (the association which regulates pet food) and the National Research Council, and to our analysis of the natural diet of dogs and cats. Our excellent data on the natural diet comes from anthropological studies and work done by zoos on the composition of prey animals.

Our food plan is designed to replicate the balance and content of the food dogs and cats really ate — mostly small prey, with some scavenging for dogs. That means that organs are included in the recipes. **Use all the ingredients or your pet will be missing some essential nutrients.** We offer some suggestions to make that part easy. For example, if you find it hard to deal with organ meats, you can buy most of them freeze dried and use them as treats. You cannot leave out the bone meal, the minerals, or the fatty acid supplements. You might look at your pet and say, "Oh, he's fine without that stuff, he looks great!" but irreversible damage may show up down the road.

Rotation is a big part of our plan. Over the course of a week, you rotate through beef, chicken, eggs, fish and turkey. You'll supply your pets with almost all of their nutrients in whole food form. The total weight of the three large recipes is no more than 36 pounds. This amount will fit into most refrigerator freezers, though there won't be much room for frozen entrees or ice cream. If your space is very limited, you could rotate through one major meat source recipe at a time, adding eggs and sardines here and there and still provide good rotation.

If you find that you're leaving things out and it's just too much trouble, you're better off with commercial frozen products or even dry food. Really. At least it's balanced and provides essential nutrients.

We're not all cut out to be full-time food preparers. If you make food for a short time and decide that you're not inclined to "cook" for your animals, following this plan even for a while will give you great insight into commercial foods and you'll be much better able to evaluate them.

The recipes as planned here have ingredients chosen partly for their energetics in Traditional Chinese Medicine; thus the beef is paired with veggies and fruits to provide a "cooling" meal, and the chicken is paired with choices to provide a "warming meal." Fish and eggs are neutral. "Food Therapy" is a very large area of study in several forms of medicine and we're providing only for the most basic of applications.

If you cook for your human family, these ideas are easy to incorporate into your routine. If you don't cook at all for yourself, after you make pet food for a while you might see the benefits and change your mind! Or you may decide that you're able to provide one meal a day of homemade food and the other meal will be commercial food. Whatever level of homemade food you can provide will be an improvement. Making food can be an enjoyable and rewarding part of life.

Our recipes are in two sizes. Large recipes can be frozen in portion sizes that are right for your pet. The small beef and poultry recipes are enough for a day for a medium size dog, or more for smaller dogs and cats. These recipes may easily be multiplied. Egg and sardine recipes are designed to be eaten the day they are prepared, or the ingredients can be spread out over the week.

The general weekly balance of our program is:

- 5 meals of chicken
- 5 meals of beef
- 2 meals of turkey
- 1 meal of eggs
- 1 meal of sardines

Three main components are discussed:

- Meat, including the organs needed
- Veggie and fruit puree
- Necessary supplements and additions

If you revise our plan and it becomes much heavier or lighter in any of its components, nutrients will be unbalanced.

There may be sound reasons to feed mostly beef, or a need to feed a novel protein diet, or a dog who right now can only tolerate one protein source.

If you have sick dogs who need limited ingredient or novel protein diets, the mineral and fat balance of this plan will not be adequate. We can help you balance a single-protein or limited ingredient diet with our consult service. Our goal will be to help you promote better health in your animal so he can eventually eat a wide variety of foods.

PREPARATION PRINCIPLES, EQUIPMENT AND STORAGE

PREPARATION PRINCIPLES

Even though dogs are built to be able to digest carrion (dead animals), their digestive systems aren't always in great shape. Dogs and cats frequently suffer from poor digestion. Both pets and humans need to be protected from toxic food. Very low levels of pathogens multiply rapidly at room temperature. Simple food preparation guidelines keep everyone safe. In cold weather it's easy to keep things cool while you make food, but in warmer weather pathogens grow quickly. The following guidelines will help keep your fresh meat safe and your produce from losing valuable phytonutrients and vitamins. Remember, you are using all "human" ingredients. There are no more bacteria on your cutting board after making "dog food" than there are after you prepare dinner for your family. Use the same common sense and disinfecting procedures for both.

Prepare food quickly to prevent meat from becoming warm and produce from losing vitamins. If you're making food for a day or two, this is easy to do, but if you're making big quantities it's more of a challenge. Refrigerate the parts you're not working with. Keep things cold! Coolers can be a great help, with a bag of ice on the bottom. Make sure you're prepared before you start.

Keep utensils and containers clean. Processing meat (or even veggies) can be a messy process! If you're making a lot of food, clean up every hour or so. Wash everything with hot soapy water, and begin again. Scrub bowls, knives, counters and food processor containers. Use common sense. The food that you're putting in that giant bowl may be cold, but if the bowl is being used for the fifth time, leftover food on the edges could be quite warm.

Food must be frozen quickly and it must be protected from air to preserve fragile nutrients. On food preparation days, get your freezer space organized so that you can spread out your containers for the fastest cooling/freezing. Stacking freezer containers tightly will result in very slow freezing. You may find unfrozen contents as much as two days later. Existing pathogens can multiply in these conditions. This is important for both meat and veggie mixes, as vitamins and phytonutrients are lost when exposed to air and light. Your freezer may have a "quick-freeze" setting — use it!

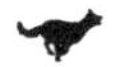

STORAGE

Good storage is essential for food safety and palatability. It's distressing to put effort, time and love into making a great batch of food and have it spoil or lose quality from poor storage. Freezer-burned food has lost nutrition, and it tastes like old ice cream or frozen pizza that fell to the bottom of the freezer for a year.

Containers must keep food protected from air. The easier they are to wash and store, the better your food preparation experience will be. Freezing food in amounts that will be used in a day makes for fast thawing and easy rotation, but for some people larger containers work well.

The ideal container for freezing is glass, which provides the best protection from air. Freezer jars have straight sides and are made from glass designed to withstand repeated freezing. These jars, which can be reused indefinitely, waste no resources and impart no plastic substances to the food. Disadvantages are that they take up a lot of storage space and are very expensive. Sizes are limited. Over time, they pay for themselves — they don't wear out.

Plastic containers range from food industry grade (expensive, long wearing and relatively non-toxic) to semi-disposable. The quality of the food industry containers is excellent, but to buy enough for two medium size dogs for a month is a hefty purchase. They nest inside each other and take up less space than glass. You can find them at restaurant supply houses and online. Semi-disposable containers, designed to hold up through about five uses, are fairly durable and last far longer than five uses. They also stack well for storage and freezing and protect food well. When they start to crack, recycle them. Plastic containers of all kinds are available in many sizes, but due to the limitations of home freezing (food doesn't cool as fast as in commercial freezing) we think that a container that holds 4 pounds is the largest container that should be used.

Plastic bags can be used, but they should be designed for the freezer. Regular bags don't do a good job of protecting food from air. Freezer bags aren't as easy to stack and store in the freezer as rigid containers and they're not easy to reuse, though it can be done. If you're storing food for a long time, even freezer bags should be double-bagged. You can store a batch of smaller bags inside one large bag and still get the protection of double bagging.

If you're really thrifty and if using plastic is ok with you, used plastic containers do a good job of protection and are sturdier than the semi-disposable ones. Cottage cheese containers, ricotta and yogurt — many containers can be reused. If all your containers are the same, storage is easier, but free is good!

Labels are a good idea. You may think that you will remember what you put in those containers and you may think that your abbreviation is perfectly clear, but trust us — it's best to label your containers clearly with enough words so that you really know what you meant. It's wise to date them while you're at it. Masking tape or freezer tape both work well.

EQUIPMENT

You can get by with almost no equipment starting out, but a few basics are needed or you'll have a big surprise trying to find a container to mix ten pounds of food.

A Really Big Bowl is needed. Stainless steel is cheap, durable and easy to find. Several very large bowls wouldn't be excessive. Plastic isn't the best choice for many reasons. Aside from the environmental reasons to avoid plastic as much as possible, most plastic bowls tend to hang on to grease. They become unpleasant to handle and hard to clean. The grease that hangs on becomes rancid — not something you want to add to your nice fresh food.

Real measuring spoons and cups help you to be accurate. For some things, this is very important. Stainless is a good choice for measuring spoons, too. If you have small animals, you need a set of tiny spoons for your mineral mix, because the measuring spoons generally available don't have spoons smaller than ¼ teaspoon. These are for measuring a serving of the vitamin/mineral supplement that you'll be adding daily. They're called "spice" or "smidgen" spoons and are easy to find online, but we haven't seen them in stores.

Dry measuring cups, which you fill and then level, give an accurate measurement for our purposes. Glass cups are easier to keep clean, but for semi-solid food it's hard to know exactly how much you have in a glass cup. Dry measuring cups are usually plastic.

Knives and cutting boards are pieces of equipment you may already have. Keep your knives sharp and use separate cutting boards for veggies and meat if you're doing both on the same day. The same sanitation requirements exist as for preparation of "human" food. A cutting board used for meat for several hours could develop some unpleasant inhabitants. Scrub and sanitize your cutting boards after use.

Gloves may be useful. Hands can get amazingly cold when you make a lot of food and after you wash your hands about twenty times they get a bit dry! Whether you choose disposable gloves or those that are more heavy duty, don't feel like a coward if gloves sound like a good idea to you.

A food scale will help you know exactly what you're doing. As you gain experience, you might be able to estimate what a pound looks like, but even the most experienced tend to drift up or down in measuring. It's good to know how much you're really feeding your animal even if you're a casual sort. Scales are inexpensive and easy to use. Set your scale to "pounds and ounces" instead of "grams and kilograms" or you'll be confused! Measurements may be done in cups but it's easy to be off by a few ounces using cups. That's a lot for a medium to small dog or a cat.

A food processor will puree your vegetables and fruits. Dogs and cats don't have the enzymes to digest the cellulose that is the cell wall of veggies and fruits, so we puree them to make it easier for the digestive process to take place (in the ancestral diet, most veggie and fruit content would be predigested). When the puree is frozen, this cell wall is further broken down by the action of water expanding as it freezes. High-powered blenders like the Vita-Mix® or a regular blender work well, but a food processor can do the job with no fuss. Organ meats are quickly chopped and pureed in the food processor for easier handling, whether you are mixing into a larger quantity of meat or freezing small portions for use in daily meals.

A coffee grinder is needed to grind capsules and tablets for your vitamin/mineral mix. These are easy to find and cost less than $20.00.

A freezer soon becomes more than a luxury for those who make their own food, unless you like "cooking" every day. Space in our houses is often in short supply, but even a very small freezer can help you be efficient and thrifty. We all know dog people who consider a crate to be a great end table — you may find that a small freezer is a good counter surface for your kitchen. However you manage it, a freezer will make your life easier. Check the temperature of your freezer regularly. It should be able to maintain 0 degrees.

A grinder is helpful for even smaller scale food production. You can throw all your meat ingredients together and grind them in no time. Food processors don't work at all for this job. If you use all boneless meats, a $100 grinder will suffice, but may not last long. Some people swear by them, but they're slow and not very powerful. You can feed your meats and organs cut up and mixed with veggies, but the veggies are more palatable mixed with ground meat. There are ways to get around the grinder issue, but a grinder makes food preparation much faster.

If you want to grind turkey necks, or take advantage of great bargains like whole turkeys or chickens, you will need a heavy-duty grinder. This is a major purchase. It's heavy. You need a place to keep it. But there's no denying that if you're making large quantities of food, a grinder really speeds things up. Check Cabela's® catalog for a starting place. A quick search on the internet will find you many opinions and options.

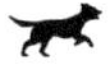

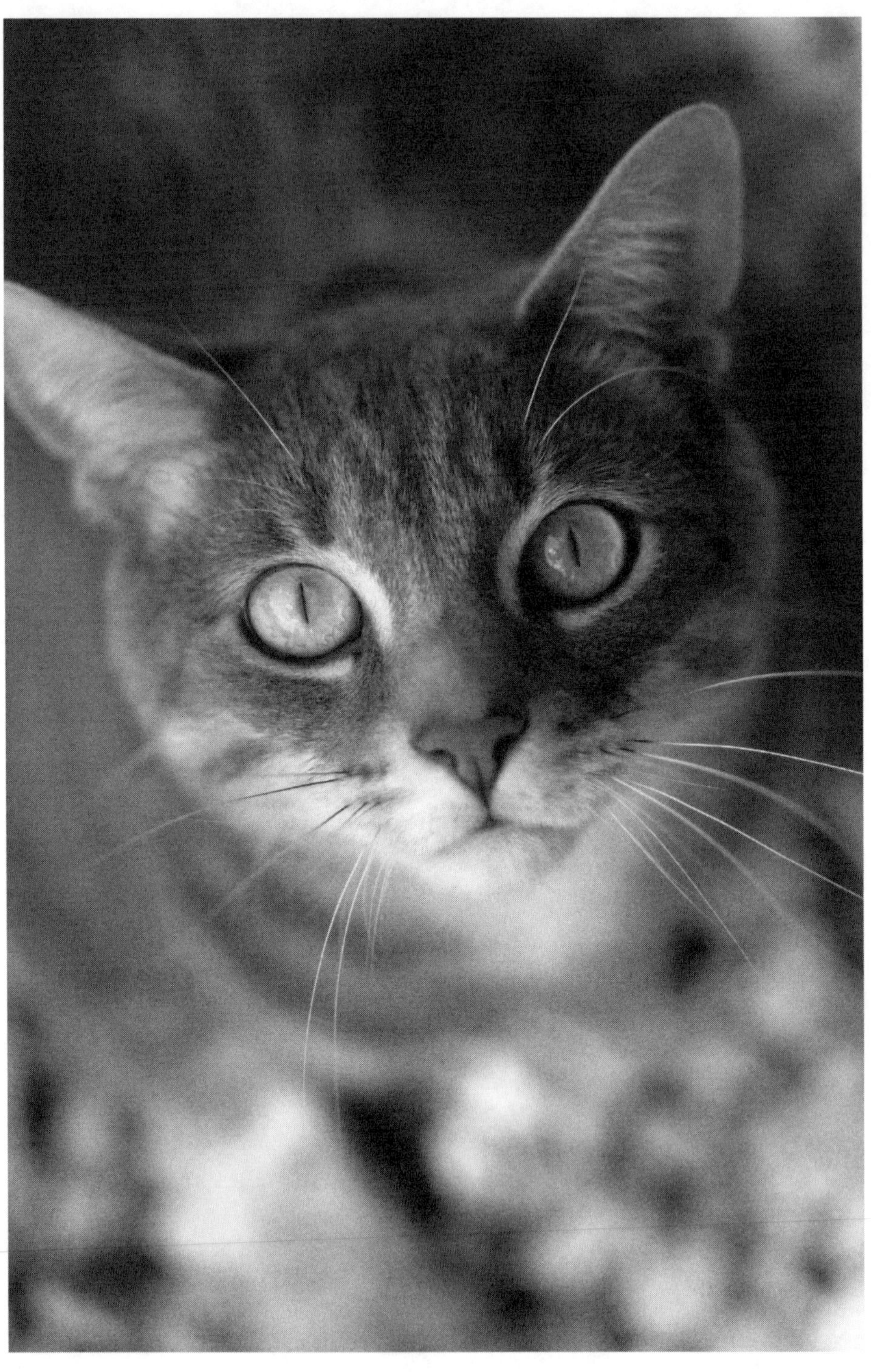

FOOD QUALITY

The meals you prepare with our plan will be superior to any commercial dry or canned food. Most dry and canned food is made from poor quality ingredients. Some are made from better ingredients, but they are still highly processed and are stored for a long time. Frozen diets may be of good quality but most are kept in cold storage at the distributor and the retailer for long periods before they get to your animal's dinner bowl. Any ingredients you buy will be fresh and significantly more nutritious.

You can make fresh, healthy food by shopping at the local supermarket or produce market, or you can make food with organic produce and grass-fed meats. The choice is yours. For very ill animals, quality is sometimes a critical factor, but there are many considerations in making this choice. You will be more critical of the quality of ingredients going into your companion's food than even the most ethical of commercial food companies.

We're for balance. We meet people who feed their animals at the very highest end of the food scale, while feeding themselves at the local fast food establishment. If you and your animals upgrade together to simply human-edible fresh food, with as little in the way of toxins as you can find in the supermarket, you'll be far ahead of where you started.

Conventional farming methods used for decades have resulted in the depletion of our soil. This means that the food we buy in our supermarkets doesn't contain the nutrients it once did. Pesticides, hormones and genetic modification of foods are very real concerns. A few shopping guidelines will be discussed in the meat section, different ones in the veggie and fruit section.

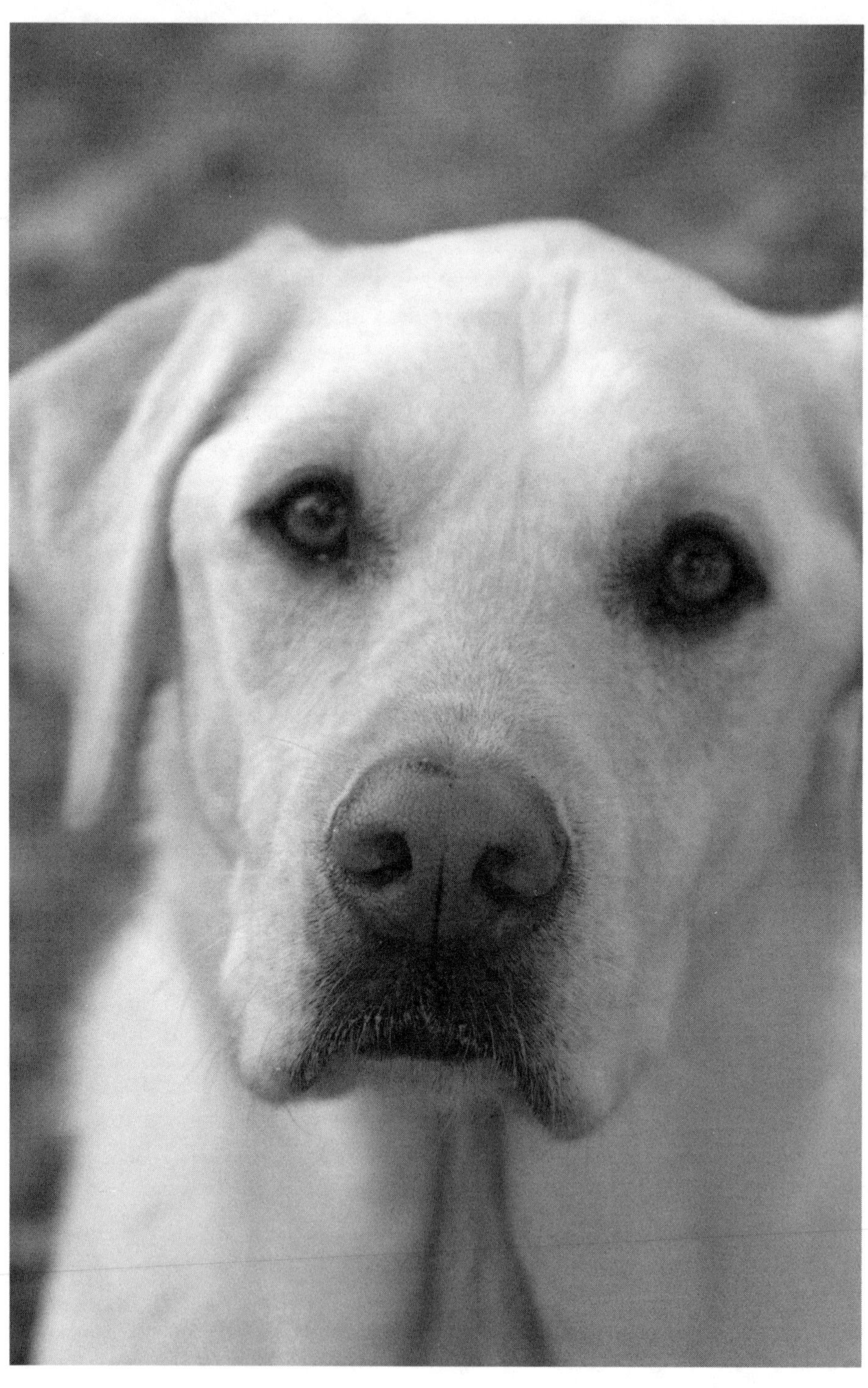

THE BIG PIECES: PROTEIN, FAT, CARBOHYDRATE AND WATER

In the ancestral diet of dogs and cats, muscle, bone and organs make up 65% – 80% of the diet of dogs, and 85% – 90% of the diet of cats. The fat content of the diet was much higher in the fall than in the spring, but averaged about 20%. This isn't a lot of fat compared to the average American diet. In dogs, dietary carbohydrates come from the gut and stomach content of small prey and from grazing and scavenging. Cats get carbohydrates from the gut and stomach content of prey (which are eaten whole) and they graze on grasses. For dogs, the carbohydrate portion might be as high as 20% or as low as 10%. Cats might average between 5% and 7%. The calorie contribution of dietary carbohydrates is very low, but the vitamin, antioxidant, phytonutrient and fiber value is high. All food contains water, a critical ingredient for digesting and absorbing food.

The balance of our program for dogs is 75% meat, organs and bone, and 25% veggies and fruit. For cats, the balance is about 88% meat, organs and bone, and 12% veggies. In our experience, this balance works for most pets.

Protein is the foundation of the diet of a carnivore, necessary for the formation of healthy cells, enzymes, hormones, ligaments, tendons, organs and protective tissue. Protein is an integral part of every cell of the body. Next to water, it makes up the majority of our pet's body weight.

The body can manufacture some of the building blocks to make the proteins it needs, but some proteins must be provided in the diet: these are the essential amino acids. Proteins help the body rebuild and repair. Organ meats provide essential vitamins and minerals.

Fat provides fuel, essential vitamins and fatty acids. Fatty acids are necessary for a host of body functions, including reproduction, normal cell membrane synthesis, normal healing and normal skin and coat. Dogs can get some of these fats from plant sources, but they do much better with animal sources. Cats, being obligate carnivores, must get certain fatty acids from meat sources. Fats are very delicate. At high temperatures or exposed to air, they become rancid rapidly. Commercial foods usually include antioxidants to protect the fats, but fat still spoils quickly. Your fresh homemade food, with lots of variety, will give your animal more fresh nutritious fats than any commercial food.

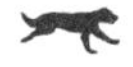

The fat level of our program is at the level of the ancestral diet (about 20% of the calories are provided by fat). We balanced the fats with the addition of krill, flax and hemp oils to make up for the differences in the meat we buy today compared to the meat that would have been the natural prey of cats and dogs.

More important information on fats can be found in *See Spot Live Longer*, available at our website and in Steve Brown's book, *The ABC Way*.

Carbohydrate in the ancestral diet of dogs and cats is limited to plants and berries, and the stomach and gut content of prey animals. We supply those carbohydrates with vitamin- and mineral-rich vegetables and fruits.

Studies over a 30 year period of wild canid and felid feces and stomach content confirm that the natural diet of these species does not include the high-carbohydrate end of the plant spectrum, grains and seeds, unless they are pre-digested by small prey animals. Dogs and cats (and many people) are not designed to cope with large quantities of these substances without long-term metabolic consequences, chronic illness and dysfunction, specifically unregulated inflammation.

You will not find rice, barley, oats or any high-carbohydrate foods in our program (except for small amounts of sweet potatoes and pumpkin). For most animals, these foods contribute to chronic inflammation and ill health.

Should an animal be in organ failure, unable to process protein, then he may need to consume more starchy vegetables like sweet potatoes or pumpkin, or even rice. These dietary alterations should be supervised by a veterinarian who has experience with fresh food diets.

Water is a dietary component we don't think about much. If your water is clean and toxin free, you're very lucky. Much urban water has chlorine and fluoride and other substances that are not desirable. For yourself and your animals, we suggest taking a look at your water. At the very least, a water filter pitcher (like a Brita®) can take some of the toxins out. Some water purifiers take out the minerals — we want to leave the minerals in the water. Bottled water may be a good answer, but many bottled waters are without minerals and others are no better than tap water. Do some research on this topic and you'll come up with a solution that will be appropriate for your life.

MEATS

Our plan is designed to include all the meats and vegetables we've given you in the recipes. The analysis was done with five meals of chicken, five meals of beef, two meals of turkey, one meal of eggs and one meal of sardines. This basic program provides good variety and balance.

We'll briefly discuss meats other than those included in the recipes so you'll have some information we think is important if you decide to use a different meat, but the minerals needed and the fat balance will change somewhat. We'll be glad to help you re-balance the nutrients.

At the grocery store level, careful shopping can reduce the cost of meat. Big box stores like Costco® and Sam's Club® regularly offer chicken at very low prices. Grocery and warehouse chain stores offer meat specials like round steak for half the regular price. Turkeys are very cheap around Thanksgiving. Produce markets and ethnic stores are good sources for reasonably priced meats and organs. Get to know the meat people — they usually love to help and can't believe that you're really making dog and cat food. They can tell you when sales are coming up or help you find exactly what you need. The trick for taking advantage of many promotions is storage. You must have room to store large quantities of food.

The meat we buy at grocery stores usually comes from animals that have been fed antibiotics and pesticide-laden feed that's inappropriate for their bodies. It's likely that there are some residues in the meat that do not promote health. However, a fresh diet from grocery store ingredients is many steps above pet food in a bag or a can, even those products at the very highest end of the spectrum of dry and canned pet foods.

In "organic" or "natural" meat purchasing, there are no bargains. There is much to learn in order to get what you think you're getting. It's beyond the scope of this little book to educate you about this big area, but as with any product, let the buyer be educated. For example, "grass-fed beef" is very trendy and better for you in a lot of ways — but "grass-fed" may not mean "grass-finished." That beef you're paying a lot for may have been "finished"

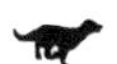

in a feedlot on grain, which means that the good fats you hope to obtain may not be there. This is just one small example. The best way to know what you're buying is to get your meat from small family farms that are concerned with good farming practices and the humane raising of food animals.

Resources abound and buying clubs exist. When you start looking you'll be amazed.

Fat contains more than twice the calories as an equal amount of protein. Room needs to be allowed in the plan for good fats — sardines, krill oil and others. When necessary fats (fish oil and other beneficial fats) are added to an already high-fat diet, the resulting caloric balance will be higher in fat than any other nutrient. If a very high fat diet is fed, there will be less room for protein in an animal's caloric allowance. If meat is higher in fat than suggested, mineral levels and other nutrients will be reduced and the natural balance of nutrients will be compromised. If your animal's liver or digestive system is overtaxed, serious problems may occur and you may see a worsening of symptoms you are trying to improve.

Buy lean meat. The fat level of the natural diet of dogs and cats varies seasonally, but it averages around 20% of the diet. Fatty beef, pork and chicken contain much more fat than the natural diet. 90-93% lean meat is what's needed to provide the optimal fat profiles found in our recipes. Check the fat content. Don't assume that you know. Turkey is usually lean, but beef is often 70% lean, 30% fat. It's no bargain to buy cheap fatty beef and drain off the fat. Ground chicken may be very high in fat. Whole meat is easier to evaluate because you can see the fat.

If you buy meat ground, it's safest to buy frozen "chubs." They have been frozen since they were packed, unlike "fresh" ground meat, which may have had inconsistent handling at the grocery store, increasing the possibility of a high bacterial load. If you are cooking, inconsistent handling is not as much of an issue. Any heavy load of pathogens will be destroyed (though their byproducts may not, and this can be a problem). Buy meat that's fresh and not close to its "sell by" date. If you become friendly with the meat people where you shop, they may grind meat to order for you.

Turkey can be found at reasonable prices in frozen one or two pound "chubs," already ground. It's usually quite lean, but check. Turkey breast and thigh are both easily found. Whole turkeys can be very affordable, especially after holidays. Organic turkeys are easy to find in regular grocery stores and turkey farmers can be found not too far from big cities. For example, close to us there is a turkey farm that sells legs, thighs and organs for the cost of cheap chicken. To make use of these bargains, you need a big grinder, as turkey bones are too big to feed whole. You can bone a turkey, but it's a lot of work, and legs are impossible to bone efficiently.

Chicken is a very cheap meat to feed your animals, but don't rely on it for the entire diet. Variety is necessary. Chicken breast is lean. Dark meat of chicken has more fat. Boneless chicken breasts and thighs are often on sale at reasonable prices — stock up on them. You may find chicken in chubs like turkey, but make sure to check the fat content — it varies a lot. If you use whole chickens, strip the fat and most of the skin before using. Strip the fat from pieces as well. The smaller the chicken, the less fat it will have. Even organic chickens often have an unhealthy layer of fat under their skin.

Beef should be at least 90% lean. That's round steak or rump roast and other lean cuts. Look for meat with very little visible fat in the muscle and remove exterior fat. Other cuts may be appropriate, but remove visible fat even from round steak if it has not been well trimmed. "USDA Select" grade meat is leaner and cheaper than "USDA Choice." There is not as much "Choice" meat in the display cases as in past years and for your pet's diet, that's a good thing. If you buy beef ground, the label will probably say "90 – 93%" lean.

Eggs (high omega-3) are a low-cost way to include beneficial fatty acids and excellent protein. In order to have good fats they need to be good eggs. Diet is the key to the superior fatty acid profiles in omega-3 eggs. For high omega-3 eggs, chickens are fed flax, which they are able to convert into more usable forms of fatty acids. For high DHA eggs, chickens are fed flax and algae, with the same good results. Better food, better chickens, better eggs. An excellent example of the benefits of real food.

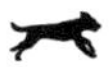

You may be able to buy eggs locally — this is always a good choice as those chickens have spent some time in the real world, outside, and are likely to have eaten some real green food. The eggs from local chickens have better nutrient content than factory farmed eggs. High omega-3 eggs, like Eggland's Best®, have good fatty acid profiles.

Feed an egg meal a week (assuming you feed your pets twice a day) or spread the amount of that egg meal over a week. If you spread the eggs out over the week just feed that much less meat mix (1.75 – 2 ounces) in those meals. Other nutrition components (fatty acids, mineral mix) won't change.

You can cook eggs lightly, but keep the yolks intact and uncooked, to protect the fragile fatty acids from exposure to air and heat.

Fish is tricky. Our program includes only sardines, to keep it simple. We're warned against eating much fish due to heavy metal contamination and there are many problems with farmed fish, yet fish is needed in the diet for variety and for fatty acids. To include other fish, you need to know much more than "open the can." Fresh fish might seem like a good idea and in a bigger book we'd probably include other fish as an option, but in this simple book we'll just take a small detour to briefly discuss some of the issues.

Canned sardines are our choice. These small fish don't live long enough to collect dangerous levels of heavy metals in their bodies. Sardines are wild, so the issues of what farmed fish eat and where they are grown are avoided. The bones in canned sardines are soft, unlike fresh fish. We've never had a problem with the bone aspect of canned sardines.

Much of the fish available to us has been farmed. Farmed fish don't eat their natural diet or live a natural life — you may be including some of the very toxins you're trying to avoid. Wild-caught fish are safest, but advertising is tricky. Even experienced label readers might assume, for example, that "from Norwegian waters" means wild-caught, but the very fine print discloses that they are farmed in Norwegian waters. Sometimes where fish are processed is not where they were caught. If farmed in China and processed in Canada, the print that says "Canada" is likely to be much larger than the print that says "origin: China." In addition, there are serious concerns about over-fishing of the earth's waters and high levels of toxic heavy metals in wild-caught fish.

If you feed salmon, it should be cooked. Some salmon carries a parasite. That parasite carries a microbe that can be fatal to dogs. Though various authors assert that freezing takes care of the problem, we have read scientific studies that say that this is not the case. Freezing kills the parasite, but bacteria often survive freezing. This parasite is mostly limited to salmon from Pacific waters, but you can't be sure. It's easy to eliminate the possibility by cooking the fish. Salmon should be wild, so that it provides the best fatty acids.

Bones in canned fish are soft, but bones in fish you cook at home are not. Remove the bones before feeding.

Fish other than sardines might not have the needed nutrients. A small snack of your tuna steak will do no harm to the balance of the diet, but regular fish meals other than what's included here would require recalculation of fats and minerals. For those who need a "fish" diet, we'll be happy to help you figure out the deficits for this unbalanced diet.

Lamb bought ground usually has a large amount of fat. Many pets don't do well on lamb. Don't feel compelled to spend a lot of money on something that may be too fatty anyway. Small amounts of lamb may be included in the rotation for any healthy dog or cat. If you find a source of homegrown lamb, use it!

Rabbit is usually available in ethnic grocery stores — it has almost certainly been frozen but check with the retailer to be sure. Never feed rabbit that has not been frozen. It is possible that very serious parasites may be present in rabbit that has not been frozen, but freezing kills the parasite. Some rabbit specialty companies sell their products frozen or fresh. Fresh rabbit sounds like a great idea, except for the possibility of parasites. *Buy rabbit frozen or freeze for 72 hours before using.*

Rabbit from raw frozen food companies is inconsistent in quality. We've seen some very fatty rabbit, which makes us wonder how they were raised. Other products are ground so coarsely that they may cause a problem for some pets. You could not feed these products cooked, which would make the problem even worse, but the large size of the raw bone pieces may be dangerous to even the healthy. If you find a good source, rabbit is a nice addition to your rotation.

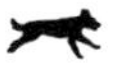

Venison is a great choice for variety. If you know hunters, they are often happy to share, particularly organ meats. Since deer aren't farm raised, they probably have lower levels of toxins than grocery store meats. We use deer organ meats, when we can get them, to upgrade the quality of a beef mix. If you can get meat *and* organs, that's even better! *As with rabbit, always freeze venison for 72 hours before using, to kill any parasites that may be present.*

Other choices include bison, ostrich, emu, goat, beaver and other exotics. Explore these possibilities if you like but don't feel that you must. You can get enough variety in what's easily found to do an excellent job.

Organ meats provide essential nutrients. Heart and liver are indispensable, vital parts of the diet. Do not skip these ingredients. We recommend higher levels of heart and liver than would be in an actual animal to make up for the missing organs and blood that we don't feed. Thus a whole chicken won't have enough heart to make up the amounts in the recipes. Chicken livers, beef liver and beef heart are readily available at ethnic grocers. You may find other body parts to include in your pet's food, too. Tripe is often promoted as a source of beneficial enzymes and people pay a lot to include it in their food programs. Tripe is useful as a low fat protein source, but unless you get it direct from the farm, enzymes have been washed away and often the tripe is bleached as well. Unless it's a bargain, it's not an important addition. Canned tripe is not a source of enzymes. Canning is a cooking process that deactivates enzymes.

Heart is a muscle meat as well as an organ. Heart contains many useful and necessary nutrients. Beef heart is easy to find and reasonably priced. Chicken and turkey are popular meat choices for most people, but poultry hearts are not as easy to find as beef. Each whole chicken usually comes with a heart, but we're including much higher amounts than the biological reality to make up for organs and blood that we don't feed.

Where heart is missing, taurine and carnitine could be added, but this covers only what we know to be needed, not the unknown. We learn daily about new nutrients in whole foods. We don't want you to use a supplement to take the place of a whole food. Stick to whole food whenever you can.

If you find heart and liver difficult to find or deal with, some commercial fresh food producers have freeze dried heart and liver available. These can be used if you're not having luck finding these ingredients, or if you'd rather not deal with the organs. You can add them to food or use them as treats. Manufacturers tell you how much freeze dried heart or liver equals one pound of fresh meat. Check the resource page on our website for sources.

Commercial frozen diet producers also offer frozen meats and organs for you to put together your own component diets.

Gizzards from chicken and turkey are often available, and usually cheap. They're very high in beneficial cartilage. Gizzards make up part of the "muscle" meat in our poultry recipes, but you can substitute an equal amount of muscle meat if you don't have gizzards.

MEAT WITH BONE

As you move through the "fresh diet" process, you may want to include bony meats. Bony meats can be good for dental hygiene and they can be a way to provide bone in its natural state. Our simple program allows for a limited amount of whole bone, as you'll see in our recipes.

Though this short book can't effectively cover the many aspects of feeding whole bone to our animals, we're including a few cautions and considerations below so you'll have a little information.

If your animal has not been weaned onto raw food, or if there are any digestive problems, take this step very slowly so you can see how it goes.

Check with your veterinarian about your dog's bite. If it is abnormal, chewing on bones may cause problems.

Exercise caution. Start after you are sure that your dog or cat is digesting raw food well. Then add whole bone slowly. If your dog is likely to swallow food whole, you may have to hold onto a chicken neck while he gnaws on it.

Feed raw bone with other food, not on an empty stomach.

The weight bearing bones of chickens, like those found in legs, are harder than necks or wings. These bones should be smashed with a heavy mallet or hammer or ground before feeding to experienced, healthy dogs who have demonstrated that they do well with raw bone. Whole birds have the proper amount of bone to meat, but few beginner pets would know how to eat them. We do not recommend weight bearing bones or whole birds for novice humans or novice pets.

Turkey necks might be appropriate for some dogs, but not for others. For example, if your Labrador takes a three pound turkey neck, crunches it twice, and swallows, this would be considered inappropriate and potentially dangerous. If he settles down and crunches slowly, that's probably ok.

Turkeys are older than chickens when they become "meat." They have used their legs and wings and their bones are harder and thicker. Turkey wings and legs are muscular, with hard bones. No turkey parts are appropriate for whole feeding except necks and those only in appropriate proportions for the dog that has handled raw bone in smaller amounts well. Turkey legs and wings and other parts are fine if they are ground up and used in proper proportions. The bone pieces are small and easily digestible and a good addition to our balanced plan.

The above short discussion is not intended to cover the topic of feeding whole bone and bone composition of the diet completely. More in-depth discussion can be found on our DVD, *Fresh Fast Food for Our Furry Friends.*

COOKED OR RAW?

Your carnivorous companion needs to eat a meat-based diet. If it can be raw, that would be best. If you can't manage the idea of raw meat, don't let that stop you from providing a homemade meat-based diet. Just cook it.

Some dogs don't like raw food or don't do well on raw food. That's ok. Their meat-based diet can be cooked. If your animal is ill, consult with your holistic veterinarian about the best way to start. Do what makes you comfortable. There are many ways to feed a fresh food diet.

If you are repulsed by the idea of feeding your animal raw meat, don't do it. If you think that raw meat is dangerous, cook the food.

Don't ever cook and feed whole bony meats (chicken necks, backs, wings, meaty bones). They become brittle and can harm your pet. If your food mix includes raw ground bone, do not cook it. If you use bone meal or other powdered calcium/phosphorus supplement, food may be cooked.

The tastes and needs of your dog or cat may change. Animals who have been happily devouring their food raw may one day refuse it. Some animals like their food warmer in the winter. Some prefer food cooked when they get older. In Traditional Chinese Medicine, there are conditions when cooked food is indicated and conditions when raw food is what's needed. We've known people whose philosophy about food led them to ignore what their animals were telling them. Be observant and flexible. Does cooking food remove vital nutrients? Yes, but a home cooked meal is still better than most of your other options.

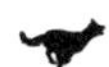

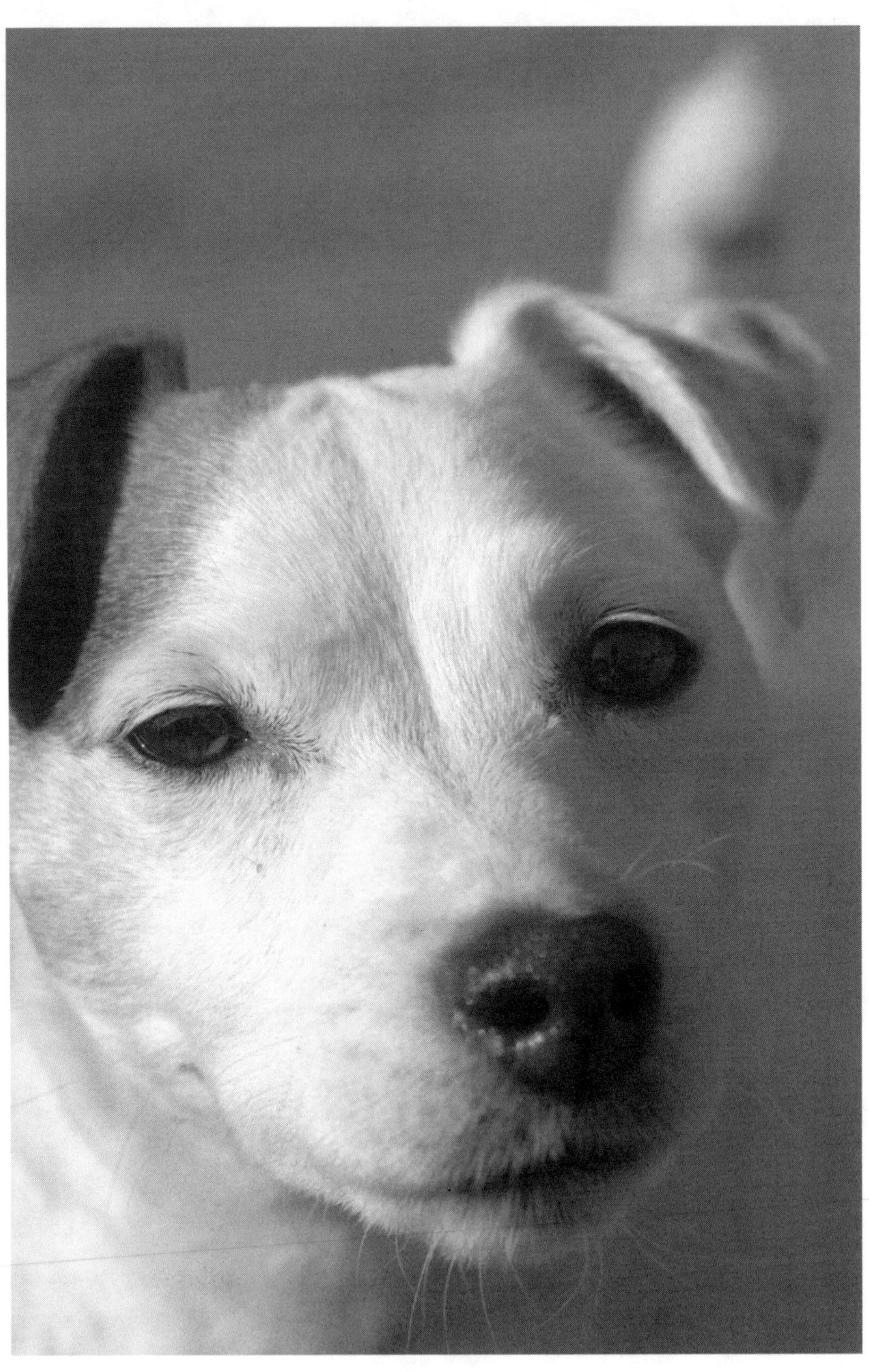

VEGETABLES AND FRUIT

What goes into your mix varies with the season. Choose what you include according to what's reasonably priced and available. Include as much variety as you can. Seasonal choices grown closer to home will be fresher than, for example, an apple from New Zealand. There's no reason to include seven kinds of expensive organic greens (unless, of course, you're eating them, too!).

Grocery store produce has plenty of pesticide and fungicide residue. Pesticide and fungicide residues are hard for the body to get rid of and they are a serious burden to the liver and kidneys. Much of this residue can be washed off. You can use a wash product designed for the purpose, you can use a very dilute solution of dish detergent with a thorough rinse — even a good rinse with plain water will remove much of the residue. Fungicides are used on potatoes and fruits. These chemicals are no better for you than pesticides and they're hard to get off. Unless you know your produce is free of fungicides, you're better off discarding the skin. The rinds of fruits are usually treated with fungicides, so discard the rinds. To be really careful, wash the fruit before cutting it open. Produce department staff can usually tell you how products have been treated, and the boxes produce is packed in are often labeled with the preservatives used.

Produce grown in the US has been subjected to lower levels of pesticides than that grown in Mexico and other countries. California standards are about the best in the country in this regard. Grocery stores are beginning to post the country of origin of their produce as the demand for this information grows.

The more color the better — red peppers have more vitamin A than green ones, for example. Orange, dark green, leafy, red — lots of color indicates lots of nutrients.

Use produce that is fairly low in calories or low on the glycemic index. Keep fruit and "below ground" vegetables (potatoes of all sorts, carrots, root vegetables) to about 10-15% of the mix. More than this will result in much more sugar or carbohydrate than is natural for a dog or cat. In one pound of veggie mix, that's only about two ounces.

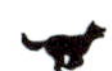

It's easy to make a big batch of veggie and fruit puree and freeze it. However, because the produce is raw, it does not have a long freezer life. Those great enzymes are slowed down but not stopped by freezing. Make what you can use in a month or two and freeze in amounts you can use within a couple of days after thawing.

Cut veggies and fruit up and puree them in a food processor, blender or Vitamix® — a little water can be added to make the process easier on the machine.

A cooked sweet potato or a can of pumpkin can be used over a period of several days. Cook sweet potatoes and winter squashes for better digestion. Canned pumpkin is simple, but lots of orange vitamins are lost in canning, so include fresh cooked sweet potatoes and pumpkin, too.

In winter, broccoli, greens, apple and carrot can be a good start. In summer there is much more variety at a reasonable price — use melons, tomatoes, zucchini and whatever looks good.

Broccoli, celery and greens (which include spinach, chard, collards, kale, endive, escarole, mustard and "mixed baby field greens") are an easy veggie mix. Zucchini, peppers, cabbage, cucumber and parsley are another.

Easily available fruits like apple, pear, orange, berries, tomatoes, pumpkin and melons of all kinds provide a wide range of nutrients. Papaya and pineapple are potent sources of the enzymes needed to help digest food, and berries of all sorts are intense blasts of antioxidants.

Green beans and all other legumes are more digestible cooked than raw. White potatoes have very little to offer — the high carbohydrate level is not offset by great nutrients, as with sweet potatoes.

Frozen vegetables may be used. They're harvested at their peak and if they've been stored well, the nutrition content is good. Eventually you will run out of variety, so use frozen vegetables in conjunction or rotation with fresh. Canned is the least nutritious choice.

Our veggie puree recipes are very specific, but you can use the information above to vary them a bit without changing the nutrient balance much. If you substitute, use similar colors and starch levels.

WHAT SHOULD YOU LEAVE OUT?

- Exclude onions and raisins. Both may cause serious problems for cats and dogs.
- Raisins may contain mycotoxins, which are a common contaminant of grapes. These toxins are harmful at very low levels. Read *See Spot Live Longer* for more on mycotoxins, one of the main contaminants of dry food. The pervasive nature of mycotoxins is a compelling reason to eliminate dry food from your pet's diet.
- Don't feed foods in the broccoli family every day. This nutritious family, the brassicas, includes kale, collards, broccoli, cauliflower, broccoli-raab, bok choy and others. If you fed (or ate) these vegetables in very large amounts every day for an extended period they could cause a problem with iodine uptake, which might impact thyroid balance. Plan a couple of days a week with nothing in your veggie mix from the broccoli family.

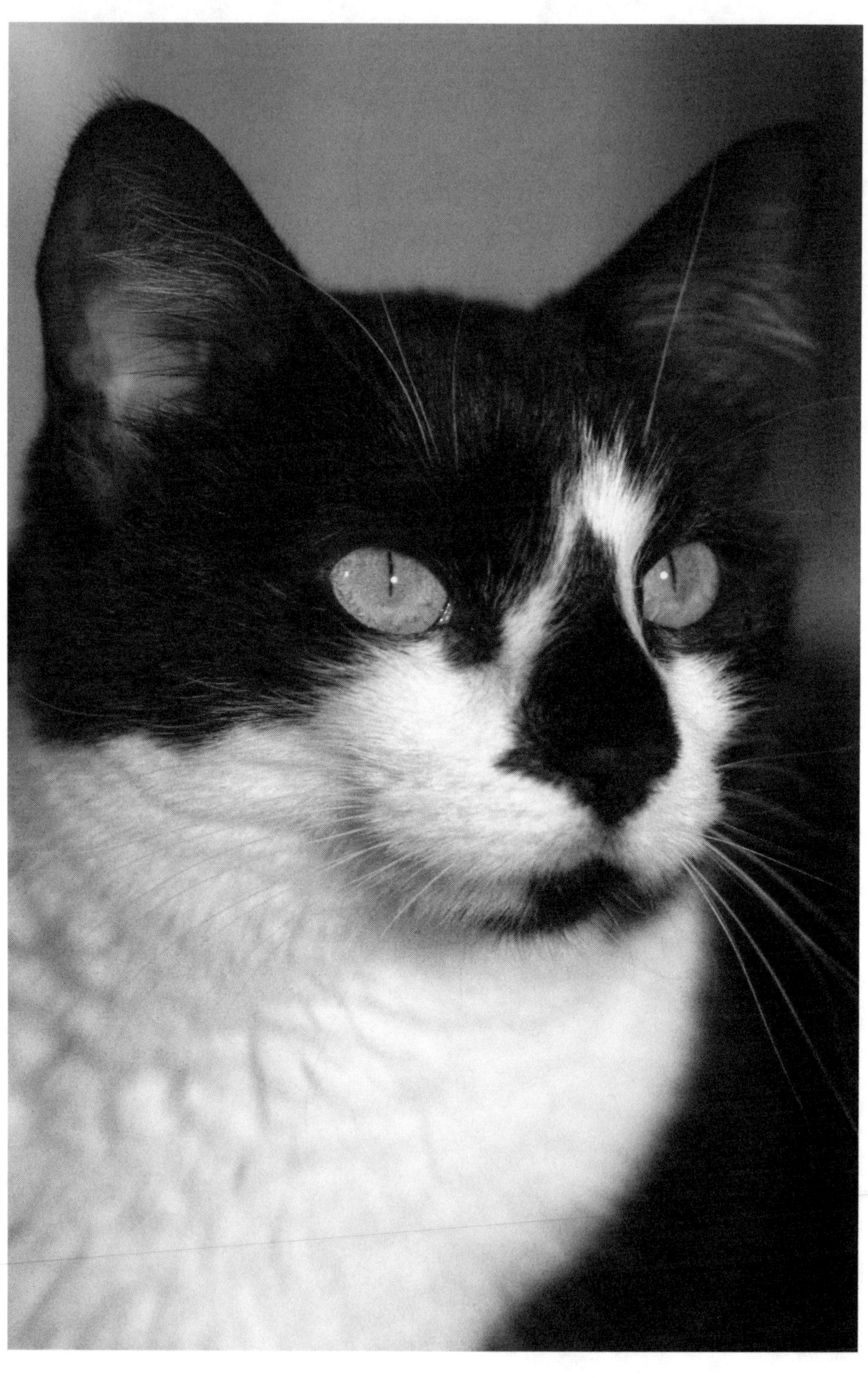

ADDITIONS

Your goal is to provide good fuel so that your pet's brilliantly designed body can do its job. Fresh food provides most of those ingredients, but some additions are needed to complete the diet. These include a bone replacement, fatty acids to balance the fats, salt and some minerals and vitamins that are in short supply in fresh foods because of the ways that we farm and raise our food animals. Non-essential but desirable additions (we think they're of great benefit to all animals) include a glandular product, enzymes and probiotics. When buying supplements, vary your products. Find a couple of brands at least and rotate through them when you can. Sometimes the acceptable choices are limited. In general, buy small quantities and try a different brand when you're ready to purchase again.

Bone in some form is necessary for proper calcium and phosphorus balance in diets that use boneless meats. We recommend two products: bone meal and MCHA. We give you amounts in recipes based on the calcium content of the bone meal. If you feed recipes with bony meats, do not add calcium.

Bone meal is ground, cooked bone. It provides the minerals of whole, raw bone without the fat and protein that come along with fresh, raw bone. Contrary to rumor, human edible bone meal made in USDA plants has a certificate that it has been tested for heavy metals and other contaminants. In order to be used by a USDA company, each batch of bone meal must have its own certificate that it passed this testing. Good pet supplement companies can sometimes document that heavy metal testing for their products has been done. It's worth noticing that Solgar® bone meal is from porcine sources, the only product that is not from beef. Usually dogs with sensitivities to beef do fine with bone meal from beef, but some do not. For these, the Solgar® bone meal is a good choice. Do not use bone meal intended for the garden.

MCHA, microcrystalline hydroxyapatite, is freeze dried bone, usually from New Zealand. It's the best quality way to provide a bone replacement. Standards for feeding in New Zealand are better than in the US. Freeze drying is not a cooking process — the bone is raw.

There is substantial variation in the amount of calcium and phosphorus in bone products. There is also considerable leeway in the amount of bone recommended by pet food regulations. We've designed our recipes around both the ancestral diet and pet food industry standards, so the amounts recommended are safe and accurate.

Below are calcium levels for some brands of bone meal we found online and in stores, so you can see the difference. Products change, so don't use the below examples for your calculations. As you can see, the amount of calcium per gram of bone meal in one product could be twice as much as another, so you need to make the effort to read the label and calculate. Make a note on the recipe page (cookbooks are meant to be written in) or make a recipe card to consult when you prepare food. Dogs and cats have different requirements. Feeding charts on each recipe page give the amount of calcium to add in grams and milligrams of calcium.

- KAL®: cooked bovine bone meal from New Zealand:
  1.5 g (1500 mg) calcium per teaspoon
- NOW®: cooked bovine bone meal from US:
  1 g (1000 mg) calcium per rounded teaspoon
- Solgar®: cooked porcine bone meal from US:
  .7 g (700 mg) per teaspoon
- MCHA: freeze dried (raw) bone from New Zealand:
  Calcium content depends on product

Dicalcium phosphate (available at some pet stores and online) may be used instead of bone meal if you prefer. Use the tables on recipe pages for the amount of calcium.

If there is a medical reason for your pet's diet to have restricted phosphorus, use calcium citrate. If your pet does not have a medical condition requiring that phosphorus be restricted, use one of the other options.

Providing the proper minerals for your home made food is one of the most important aspects of your preparation. Why would you need to supplement real food? Partly because we don't feed all the mineral- and vitamin-rich organs and blood, and partly because our farming methods have depleted the soil of minerals. Some minerals and vitamins must be added to your excellent food. Any homemade diet, however well balanced, will be short some trace minerals (usually manganese, zinc, iodine, copper and iron). In addition, cats need more thiamine and folic acid than dogs do. You could do it all with real food if you were willing to consider some odd and/or expensive ingredients, some of which your animal might not like. We don't want to make the process more complicated. Our goal is simple food.

Consider that we humans eat many foods that are fortified. We don't even think about it. Vitamin products for humans are designed to provide 100% of our needs. Dietary deficits are much less likely for us. Commercial pet foods are designed to provide 100% of dietary needs, so supplements are for specific purposes or to add a little more of some nutrients, not to supply the entire daily requirement. We've analyzed many, many supplements in the search for one that supplies the necessary pieces. Pet supplements we looked at fall very short, because they are designed as a "booster," or for a specific purpose. They may provide useful nutrients, but are lacking in proper minerals, even the ones that claim to be for homemade diets. Some recipes recommend that you use human vitamin products for dogs and cats. This seemed like a promising technique, but human needs differ from those of dogs and cats, so they don't solve the problem.

Why do so many recipes ignore this issue, or recommend human vitamins if it's not correct? We don't know. Perhaps the view is that something is better than nothing. We have read opinions from fresh food feeders that pets don't need any supplementation. We've read cookbooks which say that recipes are veterinarian approved. Most of them can't possibly provide basic nutrition. In our opinion, these people have not done their homework, and some of these ideas and recipes will ultimately do damage to the health of your animals. Just because it's written doesn't make it true. In our many years of perfecting homemade diets, analyzing diets, using dietary software and trying to find workable ways to do the job right, it's become our definite opinion that homemade diets must include the minerals and vitamins that are in short supply and they must be appropriate for the species.

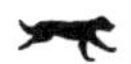

Some "nutritionists," with strong concerns that mineral and vitamin needs be met, recommend using separate products to supply each tiny need. We applaud these efforts, but it's a bit too fussy and prone to error for us. For small animals it's hard to find small enough quantities and you have to do arithmetic on a daily basis. We know you're short on time, so we give you a "recipe" to make your own mineral/vitamin powder with feeding amounts.

The vitamin, mineral and salt parts of the mix are discussed in following pages. Initially, it means you'll have to buy all the ingredients, but once you have your mix made you just add the proper amount to each meal. Because cat and dog needs are slightly different, there are two recipes.

These nutrients are essential. If you think that you're going to find this piece of the program too much to stick to, please, don't just do part of the job. Give it a try, but if it's too difficult, feed a commercial, complete food. Check our website for our upcoming commercially available "fill-in-the-gaps" powder.

Fatty acids are included in the food plan. Canned sardines and high quality eggs provide fatty acids as an integral part of their makeup. The krill, flax and hemp oils specified in the recipe additions are part of the plan, too, providing the best balance of fats for optimum nutrition. Krill oil is a source of omega-3 fatty acids. Hemp oil balances the fat in beef meals and flax oil balances the turkey and chicken. Different amounts of flax oil are needed for chicken and turkey.

Fatty acid supplements don't keep well. Take them yourself, too, and they will be used quickly. There are no bargains in oil supplements. This is an area where cheap products may be more harmful than beneficial. Use only products that can be proven to be free of heavy metal contamination. Products that have been tested are usually advertised this way. Testing information for each batch is often available on company websites. Pet product sales people may say that they have a great product, but before you buy, do some research. The same is true for human products.

Our supplement recipe includes salt, iron, copper, manganese, zinc, iodine and vitamin E. Vitamin E is a useful antioxidant and is needed to protect and process the fats in the diet. Thiamine and folate are slightly deficient for cats in our diet analysis, so they're included in the mineral supplement recipe. Taurine, an amino acid found in heart and other meats, is included in the cat supplement recipe to meet AAFCO guidelines.

Salt is low in a homemade diet. We've been told that salt is bad for us, but salt is essential in maintaining the electrical balance of the body and for many critical biological and cellular functions. In the natural diet, part of the salt would come from blood and spleen and organs we don't feed. Testing recently has showed that the iodine level in iodized salt is not reliable and would not be adequate for cats and dogs in any case. Plain salt is the base to which you add other ingredients for our nutrition powder.

Digestive Enzymes replace enzymes lost in processing and cooking, and those found in parts of prey animals we don't feed — the digestive system, where enzymes are found. There are many good products. Often, a major improvement in health and digestion is seen when enzymes are added to the diet, even when this is the only diet change.

Products with a lactose base may cause trouble for some animals. Those with "allergies" or yeast infection and Leaky Gut Syndrome, or any of the wide array of digestive difficulties, should be fed an enzyme product that is not fungal in nature. Many enzyme products are grown on a base of *aspergillus* mold. Dogs and cats with these problems are likely to be sensitive to the remains of the *aspergillus*. Use a product that includes pancreatin, which provides enzymes from pancreas, replacing some of the pancreas of prey which would be eaten if whole animals were consumed.

Enzyme products are also used therapeutically for inflammatory conditions and some medical conditions. These applications should be supervised by a veterinarian.

Probiotics nurture the balance of beneficial organisms in the gut. The best probiotics are found in the refrigerated case in your local whole food grocery or health food store. Do some research on what's available to you and consult with the trained personnel at your store. A probiotic is helpful after antibiotic use, after illness or if your animal has a chronic digestive or immune problem. The need for a probiotic is much less if you have a healthy animal who gets outside and who eats a wide variety of foods. A healthy gut maintains a good balance of micro-organisms on its own.

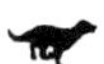

Kefir and yogurt can be included regularly in your animal's diet to provide beneficial organisms. Use plain kefir and yogurt. Don't use "diet" or "light" products. Artificial sweeteners don't belong in anyone's diet. Kefir is a better choice, because it has a wider range of beneficial organisms than yogurt.

Fiber may be needed because we don't feed our animals fur and other non-digestible sources of fiber. If your pet has dry, crumbly stools or difficulty defecating, add fiber. Ground psyllium is one of the easiest ways to add insoluble fiber if needed, but often more pumpkin or veggies will take care of a problem.

Dog's Weight	**5#**	**10#**	**25#**	**40#**	**50#**	**75#**	**100#**
Ground Psyllium	¼ t	½ t	½ t	¾ t	1 t	1¼ t	1½ t

Cats: ¼ t per cat should be sufficient

Probiotics and supplemental fiber both promote healthy organisms in the gut. However, the best way to promote healthy digestion is the easy way — eat real food and use probiotics when needed.

Glandular products are made up of all the tiny glands and organs that we are not able to supply to our animals. The internal organs and glands are components of the natural diet that are missing in almost all diets, both human and animal. They include (in addition to the heart and liver we are able to provide) pituitary, hypothalamus, adrenal, pancreas, spleen and other substances. Thyroid is classified as a drug, so if thyroid is included in a glandular product, the thyroid hormone has been removed. Glandulars are available in capsule and powder form to be added to food.

We include heart and liver in planning a diet — they're fairly easy to find. The other parts of a whole prey animal are beyond our reach (unless you become truly dedicated). To support organ systems and the function of the whole body, it may be of great benefit to include a glandular product. Check www.mypetsfriend.com for glandular products for your pet.

TREATS

What would life be like without treats?

There are many excellent commercial meat-based treats. A really good treat costs more per pound than actual food! Sometimes the cost is more than $15.00 per pound even for grocery store choices. In the "natural" pet food aisles, prices shoot toward $30.00 per pound. When reeling from the thought of the increase in cost to feed a pet fresh food, owners often forget that they're paying some seriously steep prices for treats. "Holistic" treats are very expensive. Save them for a special occasion and you might find you have more to spend on food. However, commercial treats are hard to resist, so here are a few guidelines for choosing:

- Read the very, very small print on packages. Some treats are made from ingredients purchased in China or other countries, even though they say "made in the USA." Treats made from US ingredients are less toxic.
- Watch for hidden sources of sugar: cane juice, molasses, honey, brown sugar and fructose are only a few possibilities to exclude from your acceptable choices.
- Buy treats that are made of meat only. Labels are tricky, so learn the language. Meat treats with veggies are available, but often include high-starch ingredients. Read labels carefully.
- Don't buy treats with wheat flour, white flour, oat flour, oats, barley, millet, quinoa or basically any grain ingredients. Some high-carbohydrate treats cause less intestinal havoc than others, but none are necessary or desirable — except they're really cute. Choose the "no gluten" ones and minimize their use.
- We know people with 20 different open bags of treats, they just have so much fun buying them — but with this many open bags, spoilage is an issue. Most treats (meat or grain) are best stored in the freezer.
- Cats often vote for freeze dried nuggets of fish.

Dogs (and many cats) don't care if their treats come out of a cute, expensive package. Meat is pretty popular. So are fruit and small amounts of cheese and other goodies to be found in your refrigerator (raw almonds, cashews, brazil nuts, blueberries, frozen peas — to name just a few!).

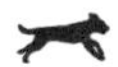

"Use small amounts" is a concept that must be learned by most of us. Small for a little dog or a cat would be a ⅛ inch square. Small for a bigger dog might be ⅛ inch to ¼ inch. We love to give treats, but they can add up to enough volume and food value to really unbalance a diet. One way to indulge yourself and your dog is to use all or part of the animal's daily food as treats. This isn't as easy to do with a fresh food diet as with dry food, but it can be done, for at least part of the ration. You can use less meat in your meat and veggie mix and save part of it for treats. You can use your organ meats as treats, making sure that you are including the full amount (and not a whole lot more) that's needed. Freeze dried organs are great for this, cut into small pieces. You can use veggies and fruits with low calorie value but high vitamin and antioxidant value, a blueberry or a piece of ripe pepper, or Dr. Becker's favorite treat, frozen peas!

Keep track of what you're handing out for a week or a day to evaluate whether you need to revise. If you're training, you may be feeding more treats than you think. Take a close look at everything you use for treats. You may be handing out some "goodies" that are not very good for your pet. There are countless great choices and for most pets, room for the occasional bakery treat. But in that case, share your pizza and forego the carbohydrate-based calorie-rich "barkery" item.

RECIPES

The first recipe in this section is for the vitamin/mineral supplement needed to provide nutrients in short supply in a fresh food diet.

The large food recipes make about 12 pounds of food for dogs or 11 pounds of food for cats (veggie content differs). This is a manageable amount to prepare and store. This amount provides food for a medium size dog for about seven to ten days, assuming that the dog eats about 1.25 pounds per day. If you have smaller dogs, it might last ten days (small dogs burn more food for their size, generally) or more. However, meat will not last that long in the refrigerator. Food that can't be used in a few days must be frozen. If you'd rather do the whole thing on a daily basis, or you have very small animals, the smaller recipes will suit you better. A small recipe provides one day's food for most medium size dogs.

Organ meats provide essential nutrients. They are mixed in with the muscle meat. The fragrance and texture of liver isn't very popular with most humans, so we think it's easier and more pleasant to mix liver and heart into a large amount of food than to deal with a daily preparation event. You could prepare organs in portion sizes and add them as you go. The variations in food preparation are infinite. Some organ meats are hard to find, though as you get more experienced you will find sources. If you can't find chicken heart or turkey heart and liver, you can buy freeze dried organs online from Companion Natural Pet Food or Bravo. These companies give you the fresh and freeze dried weight equivalents.

Meat may be cut up or ground. Organ meats may also be cut rather than ground, but it's easier to mix everything evenly if you chop the organs into pieces and chop them smaller in the food processor. Some pets do better with their organ meats pureed than with whole pieces. For example, one of our dogs regurgitates large pieces of heart but has no problem when they're ground. There is some benefit to having meat in chunks for cats and for dogs who are inclined to chew rather than gulp (no benefit for gulpers). Good for both for dental hygiene and exercise, chewing and shearing meat is a very satisfying experience for carnivores!

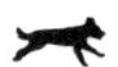

Food grinders for boneless meat can be found for around $100, but if you have a lot of dogs or big dogs, grinding meat is asking a lot of a machine that size. The big grinders are expensive, but over time, they more than pay for themselves in good, cheap food.

Recipes with bone meal or other calcium/phosphorus powder may be cooked lightly if that is your preference. A meal or a batch can be gently baked or simmered just until the meat changes color. That's enough!

DO NOT COOK RECIPES WITH RAW GROUND BONE.

For recipes with raw bone, you may substitute whole ground birds for the combined bony meats and boneless meats. This is usually the cheapest version, but requires the purchase of a large grinder.

The veggies and fruits chosen for these recipes are consistent with the food energetics of Traditional Chinese Medicine, which classifies foods as "hot/warm" or "cold/cool." The beef is a cooling meal, the chicken warming, fish and eggs neutral. We have used very simple guidelines to allow readers or practitioners to customize with more specifically therapeutic foods and herbs (please get veterinary input about diagnosis for your animal). There's much disagreement about turkey, so evaluate each case individually. For healthy animals, balance and a rotation of all ingredients is desired.

The veggie and fruit ingredients may be varied, but don't increase the starchy vegetables much, because you will add carbohydrate and change the nutrition profile.

The average calorie count of our recipes is at the low end of the range for fresh food diets, averaging about 35-40 calories per ounce. The reason for this is the fat balance. We've kept the percentage of calories coming from fat to that of the seasonal average of the ancestral diet. For bigger animals, small changes in volume don't make a huge difference. You can adjust as you go with our feeding chart. For small dogs and cats it can be very important to know how many calories you're feeding. For example, an eight pound mature cat needs about 240 calories a day, so it's easy to figure out that this cat needs about 6-7 ounces of food. An ounce is only about 2 tablespoons of food. With a small animal, a little more or a little less counts more!

You can mix your meat, organs and veggies together, or you can prepare them separately and mix together at the time of feeding. The options we offer are just starting places and you'll find ways that work for you. Meat keeps better long-term (more than a couple of months frozen) than produce. If you are making a large quantity of food, it's probably best to store the meat mix and veggie puree separately. The enzymes in the veggies and fruit will continue to act — slowly — because the food is raw. Veggie puree stored more than a month or two will lose flavor and quality due to this action.

Krill oil and other perishable additions are best added at meal times. Additions like psyllium or pumpkin might be added for a specific purpose but not on a daily basis, so they should also be added at the time of feeding, as needed.

SOME TERMS AND ABBREVIATIONS

To accurately measure cups, ingredients must be chopped, pureed or ground first and then mixed. Or, you can weigh everything on a food scale and mix and puree it all afterward. Whatever works for you is fine. Small amounts and additions given as "teaspoons" (t) or "Tablespoons" (T) are small enough quantities to be accurate and need not be weighed.

For cups, use dry measure cups. When they are filled and leveled, the volume will be very close to the weight desired.

For really small oil quantities like ¼ teaspoon or less, it's easy and less messy to use a dropper bottle. Oils are in small quantities for small animals. A little experimentation will tell you how many drops of your product equal ¼ or ⅛ teaspoon.

Just in case you think our measuring details are moving toward the obsessive, we'll add two totally imprecise terms! "Scant" means "a little less than." It's hard to be precise when using cups for small quantities, but that "little less than" adds up for small animals. In the same category is "plus." "1 c plus" means a level measuring cup that's a little rounded. Again, this may be only a tablespoon more, but it might be important to a small animal. To save space, we sometimes refer to "plus" as "+".

t = level measuring teaspoon

T = level measuring tablespoon

c = level measuring cup

= pound (16 oz)

oz = ounce

g = gram

1# = 16 oz (ounces) = 2 c

½# = 8 oz (ounces) = 1 c

If you have small animals, invest in what are labeled as "smidgen measuring spoons." These spoons measure smaller amounts than ¼ teaspoon and are needed for the mineral supplement for cats and dogs that eat less than 1 cup of food per meal. They're inexpensive and easy to find online, but we didn't find them in any stores. The spoons we have don't have the actual measurement on them, aside from "smidgen," "pinch" and "dash," so below are the equivalents.

⅛ t = a dash

1/16 t = a pinch

1/32 t = a smidgen

VITAMIN/MINERAL MIX

This recipe is one of the foundations of our program. You can shift veggies and fruits around a bit, you can vary meats, but you can't do without this mix. We chose the level of each nutrient in this recipe by reviewing pet food industry standards, analyzing the ancestral diet, and analyzing and adjusting our recipes. Specific minerals do specific jobs and they work together. Because iodine is needed for thyroid function and zinc is needed for good skin, it does not follow that more of either is better! The balance of minerals is very important. Once you have this vitamin/mineral supplement on your shelf, you can feel confident that if you follow our recipes your food will supply all the nutrients your pet needs.

Salt is the base of the supplement. Why salt? Isn't it healthier to limit salt? In the ancestral diet, blood and organs contribute substantial amounts of salt. To meet NRC and AAFCO guidelines as well as ancestral levels, salt is needed. To the salt, we add ground up vitamin and mineral tablets and capsules. A coffee grinder does a great job of grinding capsules or tablets. Other machines we tried didn't do very well.

After you count out and grind up the mineral and vitamin additions, the components are mixed and ground again briefly to make sure all the pieces are the same size, so that they stay mixed. Stir the mixture periodically, as particles are of different weights and some things may settle to the bottom of the jar.

In our recipe, we've used forms and potencies of vitamins and minerals that are easy to find and reasonably priced. If you use the same products, your results will be close to identical. The supplement amounts listed in the recipe charts are for our recipe. If you change the forms or potencies, you'll change the dose and possibly the balance. Best to do it the way we have it written.

Salt

Use salt that does not contain iodine. Iodized salt is inconsistent in its iodine content. To make sure the levels are correct, we use plain salt and add iodine from kelp. Salts like Celtic sea salt and Himalayan sea salt provide tiny amounts of trace minerals that may be beneficial. Use them if you wish, but plain table salt or sea salt is fine.

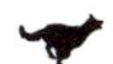

Iron

We used 18 mg Chelated Iron Biglycinate capsules from NOW® foods.

Copper

Copper is needed in very small amounts. We used Twinlabs® Chelated Copper 2 mg capsules. Copper is often sold in combination with zinc, but the balance is not appropriate. Purchase these two minerals separately.

Manganese

This mineral is sold in 10, 20 and 50 mg doses. We used Twinlabs® 10 mg Chelated Manganese capsules.

Zinc

We used NOW® 50 mg Zinc Picolinate capsules. Some individuals in some breeds have difficulty assimilating zinc. If it is recommended that your pet receive more than the normal level of zinc, add the extra amount to the food, not to the supplement recipe. Additions to the supplement recipe would affect the balance and serving size of the supplement.

Iodine

Iodine from kelp is easy to find, but you must buy a product that's standardized, not just dry kelp. In dry kelp products, iodine content can vary enough so that you might have not enough — or far too much. We used NOW® iodine from kelp, which provides 150 mcg iodine per tablet.

Vitamin E

We used NOW® "dry E" 400 iu capsules for simplicity, rather than vitamin E oil. When mixed with the other ingredients in the amount indicated, your pet will get the level we recommend daily for its weight automatically.

The additions above cover the vitamins and minerals needed for dogs.

Cats need a few additional nutrients. They're obligate carnivores, not scavenging carnivores and the recommendations of regulatory agencies reflect that difference. Use separate mixes for dogs and cats.

Taurine

The taurine included in the recipe for cats is at the level recommended by AAFCO. While fresh food diets have considerable taurine, various factors can influence these levels. Include taurine in your mix. We used NOW® 1 g Taurine capsules.

Thiamine and Folate

Two parts of the B vitamin complex, thiamine and folate, need to be supplemented in a fresh food diet for cats. Though the amounts are small, to meet nutrition recommendations they must be included. We used NOW® 100 mg B-1 (thiamine) and NOW® Folic Acid 800 mcg tablets.

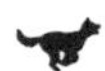

Vitamin mineral supplement for dogs — enough for 190 pounds of food

¼ c	plus	salt (72 g)
56	capsules	iron chelate 18 mg capsules (we used NOW®)
58	capsules	copper chelate 2 mg capsules (we used Twinlabs®)
10	capsules	manganese chelate 10 mg capsules (we used Twinlabs®)
20	capsules	zinc 50 mg capsules (we used NOW® picolinate)
136	tablets	kelp — 150 mcg tablets natural iodine (we used NOW®)
25	capsules	vitamin E 400 iu capsules (we used NOW® "dry" vitamin E)

Vitamin mineral supplement for cats — enough for 170 pounds of food

¼ c	plus	salt (72 g)
41	capsules	iron chelate 18 mg capsules (we used NOW®)
110	capsules	copper chelate 2 mg capsules (we used Twinlabs®)
16	capsules	manganese chelate 10 mg capsules (we used Twinlabs®)
5	capsules	zinc 50 mg capsules (we used NOW® picolinate)
43	tablets	kelp — 150 mcg tablets natural iodine (we used NOW®)
25	capsules	vitamin E 400 iu capsules (we used NOW® "dry" vitamin E)
20	capsules	taurine 1 g capsules (we used NOW®)
1	tablet	thiamine 100 mg tablets (we used NOW® B-1)
11	tablets	folate 800 mcg tablets (we used NOW® folic acid)

This isn't a general supplement. It's been designed for our proportions of meat and veggies and fruits; one version for cats, and one version for dogs. If you use different recipes, the mineral supplementation might look quite different. For example, higher fat recipes would require different mineral levels. Evaluation of the ingredients would be needed to determine the correct levels.

Recipes that don't include some supplemental mineral ingredients are unlikely to meet the nutrition requirements of your animal. You may not see symptoms of deficiency. But over time, the lack of necessary nutrients will have a negative impact on many functions of the body.

Our desire is to help you create abundant health through the best home-made diet available. Please follow these instructions and do not exclude any ingredients.

Be aware that this is a dusty procedure. Go slowly and avoid stirring things up too much. Dust can be irritating to the respiratory system!

Measure the salt into a small bowl big enough to mix everything together.

Count out all your capsules and tablets. Grind them in small batches in a coffee grinder, in bursts of a few seconds at a time to prevent heat buildup. The gelatin from capsules could melt if you grind long enough to heat up the mix. Too little or too much in a coffee grinder changes how well the machine can work. We've included the capsules for simplicity — if you take the contents out of the capsules and discard the capsules you'll change the end product — so just grind them all up. Sift large capsule pieces out after everything is ground up.

Add the mineral-vitamin powder to the salt and stir.

Then grind this mix again, in batches that fit in the coffee grinder to make sure all the particles are as close to the same size as they can be.

Keep the powder in a closed, moisture proof container like a screw-top glass jar. It's a good plan to fill a small jar to work out of if you have small animals, so the larger amount doesn't get contaminated by food. This may seem like a needless precaution, but putting together meat and veggies at mealtime can be sloppy event.

If you have lots of animals, it might be worthwhile to multiply the quantities and make more than one batch at a time.

That's all there is to this procedure! The importance is in the ingredients. Every ingredient is included in the balance and amount that will provide optimum nutrition to your diet program.

The different ingredients included in the cat supplement would not be harmful for dogs, but they have not been proven to be essential, and the recommendations for some ingredients are quite different for cats and dogs. Make both varieties if you have cats and dogs.

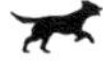

Boneless beef, large recipe – Feed 5 beef meals a week

A BEEF MEAL = Meat Mix + Veggie Puree + Bone Supplement + Mineral/Vitamin Mix + Krill + Hemp

• Meat mix for dogs or cats

8.5#	(17 c) beef, 90-93% lean
1#	(2 c) beef heart
8 oz	(1 c) beef liver

Grind or chop meat and organs. Mix meat and organs well.

• Veggie and fruit puree for large recipe boneless beef

For dogs		For cats	
1.5#	(3 c) broccoli	11.5 oz	(scant 1 1/3 c) broccoli
13 oz	(1 2/3 c) celery	6.5 oz	(¾ c +) celery
11 oz	(1 1/3 c +) blueberries	5.5 oz	(2/3 c) blueberries
6 oz	(¾ c) watermelon	3 oz	(¼ c +) watermelon

Wash produce and drain. Chop roughly and puree in batches your blender or food processor can handle, with a little water as needed.

• Combine meat mix with veggie puree

There are two ways to combine meat mix with veggie puree.

1. Combine the entire meat mix recipe with the entire veggie puree recipe for your species. Proportions of meat and veggies will be correct.
2. Freeze veggie puree and meat mix separately and mix at time of feeding.

Below are proportions for combining meat and veggies after thawing.

Meat mix to veggie puree proportions for cats and dogs

DOGS 3 parts meat mix to 1 part veggies = 3 c meat mix + 1 c veggies
CATS 7 parts meat mix to 1 part veggies = 7/8 c meat mix + 1/8 c veggies

Freeze in convenient amounts to use within a day or two after thawing.

• Add supplements at mealtimes

Add calcium source (bone replacement), mineral/vitamin mix and both oils at mealtimes, using the tables below. *Amounts given for all supplements are for meat mix with veggie puree added.*

Add enzymes, glandular, probiotics and other supplements at mealtimes as well, using product guidelines.

Bone supplement providing specified amount of calcium

Cups fed	Dog		Cat	
¼ c	.27 g	(275 mg)	.19 g	(188 mg)
½ c	.5 g	(535 mg)	.37 g	(375 mg)
1 c	1 g	(1000 mg)	.75 g	(750 mg)
2 c	2 g	(2142 mg)	1.4 g	(1413mg)
3 c	3.2 g	(3200 mg)	2.1 g	(2100 mg)
4 c	4.2 g	(4300 mg)	2.8 g	(2800 mg)
5 c	5.3 g	(5355 mg)		
6 c	6.4 g	(6426 mg)		
7 c	7.5 g	(7500 mg)		
8 c	8.6 g	(8568 mg)		

Mineral/vitamin mix – Dog and cat servings are the same, but formulas are different

Cups fed	Dog	Cat
¼ c	1/32 t	1/32 t
½ c	1/16 t	1/16 t
1 c	⅛ t	⅛ t
2 c	¼ t	¼ t
3 c	⅜ t	⅜ t
4 c	½ t	½ t
5 c	½ t +	
6 c	¾ t	
7 c	¾ t +	
8 c	1 t	

Fatty acid supplements for beef: use BOTH hemp and krill oil

Cups fed	Hemp Oil	Krill Oil
¼ c	4 drops	35 mg
½ c	7 drops	75 mg
1 c	½ t	125 mg
2 c	1 t	250 mg
3 c	1 ½ t	375 mg
4 c	2 t	500 mg
5 c	2 ½ t	625 mg
6 c	2 ¾ t	750 mg
7 c	1 T	1000 mg
8 c	3 ½ t	1125 mg

Boneless chicken, large recipe – Feed 5 chicken meals a week

A CHICKEN MEAL = Meat Mix + Veggie Puree + Bone Supplement + Mineral/Vitamin Mix + Krill + Flax

• Meat mix for dogs or cats

7.5# (15 c) lean chicken thighs or breasts with some skin (not all the skin!)

1# (2 c) chicken heart (or equivalent amount freeze dried chicken heart)

½# (1 c) chicken liver

1# (2 c) chicken gizzards (if you don't use gizzards use 1# more meat)

Boneless chicken thighs and breasts are often on sale. They can save you a lot of work. If your pieces still have the bone in, weigh or measure after boning. Grind or chop meat and organs. Mix well.

• Veggie and fruit puree for large recipe boneless chicken

For dogs		For cats	
1#	(2 c) carrots	8 oz	(1 c) carrots
1#	(2 c) Chinese cabbage (napa)	8 oz	(1 c) Chinese cabbage (napa)
1#	(2 c) red or orange peppers	8 oz	(1 c) red or orange peppers
8 oz	(1 c) cantaloupe	4 oz	(½ c) cantaloupe

Wash produce and drain. Chop roughly and puree in batches your blender or food processor can handle, with a little water as needed.

• Combine meat mix with veggie puree

There are two ways to combine meat mix with veggie puree.

1. Combine the entire meat mix recipe with the entire veggie puree recipe for your species. Proportions of meat and veggies will be correct.
2. Freeze veggie puree and meat mix separately and mix at time of feeding.

Below are proportions for combining meat and veggies after thawing.

Meat mix to veggie puree proportions for cats and dogs

DOGS 3 parts meat mix to 1 part veggies = 3 c meat mix + 1 c veggies

CATS 7 parts meat mix to 1 part veggies = 7/8 c meat mix + 1/8 c veggies

Freeze in convenient amounts to use within a day or two after thawing.

• Add supplements at mealtimes

Add calcium source (bone replacement), mineral/vitamin mix and both oils at mealtimes, using the tables below. *Amounts given for all supplements are for meat mix with veggie puree added.*

Add enzymes, glandular, probiotics and other supplements at mealtimes as well, using product guidelines.

Bone supplement providing specified amount of calcium

Cups fed	Dog		Cat	
¼ c	.27 g	(275 mg)	.19 g	(188 mg)
½ c	.5 g	(535 mg)	.37 g	(375 mg)
1 c	1 g	(1000 mg)	.75 g	(750 mg)
2 c	2 g	(2142 mg)	1.4 g	(1413mg)
3 c	3.2 g	(3200 mg)	2.1 g	(2100 mg)
4 c	4.2 g	(4300 mg)	2.8 g	(2800 mg)
5 c	5.3 g	(5355 mg)		
6 c	6.4 g	(6426 mg)		
7 c	7.5 g	(7500 mg)		
8 c	8.6 g	(8568 mg)		

Mineral/vitamin mix – Dog and cat servings are the same, but formulas are different

Cups fed	Dog	Cat
¼ c	1/32 t	1/32 t
½ c	1/16 t	1/16 t
1 c	⅛ t	⅛ t
2 c	¼ t	¼ t
3 c	⅜ t	⅜ t
4 c	½ t	½ t
5 c	½ t +	
6 c	¾ t	
7 c	¾ t +	
8 c	1 t	

Chicken fatty acid supplement – amounts differ for turkey and chicken - use both oils!

Cups fed	Flax Oil	Krill Oil
¼ c	4 drops	35 mg
½ c	⅛ t	75 mg
1 c	¼ t	125 mg
2 c	½ t	250 mg
3 c	1 t	375 mg
4 c	1 ½ t	500 mg
5 c	1 ¾ t	625 mg
6 c	2 t	750 mg
7 c	2 ½ t	1000 mg
8 c	2 ¾ t	1125 mg

Boneless turkey, large recipe – Feed 2 turkey meals a week

A TURKEY MEAL = Meat Mix + Veggie Puree + Bone Supplement + Mineral/Vitamin Mix + Krill + Flax

• Meat mix for dogs or cats

7.5#	(15 c) boneless turkey breast or thigh meat
½#	(1 c) turkey liver (or equivalent amount of freeze dried turkey liver)
1#	(2 c) turkey heart (or equivalent amount of freeze dried turkey heart)
1#	(2 c) turkey gizzards (if you don't use gizzards use 1# more meat)

Turkey thighs and breasts are often on sale and can be great bargains. If your pieces have bone, weigh or measure after boning. Grind or chop meat and organs. Mix meat and organs well.

• Veggie and fruit puree for large recipe boneless turkey

For dogs		For cats	
1 ½#	(3 c) zucchini	12 oz	(1 ½ c) zucchini
7 oz	(7/8 c) apple	3.5 oz	(scant ½ c) apple
1 ½#	(3 c) cooked sweet potato	10 oz	(¾ c) cooked sweet potato
4 oz	(½ c) papaya	2 oz	(¼ c) papaya

Wash produce and drain. Skin sweet potato. Chop roughly and puree in batches your blender or food processor can handle, with a little water as needed.

• Combine meat mix with veggie puree

There are two ways to combine meat mix with veggie puree.

1. Combine the entire meat mix recipe with the entire veggie puree recipe for your species. Proportions of meat and veggies will be correct.
2. Freeze veggie puree and meat mix separately and mix at time of feeding.

Below are proportions for combining meat and veggies after thawing.

Meat mix to veggie puree proportions for cats and dogs

DOGS 3 parts meat mix to 1 part veggies = 3 c meat mix + 1 c veggies
CATS 7 parts meat mix to 1 part veggies = 7/8 c meat mix + 1/8 c veggies

Freeze in convenient amounts to use within a day or two after thawing.

• Add supplements at mealtimes

Add calcium source (bone replacement), mineral/vitamin mix and both oils at mealtimes, using the tables below. *Amounts given for all supplements are for meat mix with veggie puree added.*

Add enzymes, glandular, probiotics and other supplements at mealtimes as well, using product guidelines.

Bone supplement providing specified amount of calcium

Cups fed	Dog	Cat
¼ c	.27 g (275 mg)	.19 g (188 mg)
½ c	.5 g (535 mg)	.37 g (375 mg)
1 c	1 g (1000 mg)	.75 g (750 mg)
2 c	2 g (2142 mg)	1.4 g (1413mg)
3 c	3.2 g (3200 mg)	2.1 g (2100 mg)
4 c	4.2 g (4300 mg)	2.8 g (2800 mg)
5 c	5.3 g (5355 mg)	
6 c	6.4 g (6426 mg)	
7 c	7.5 g (7500 mg)	
8 c	8.6 g (8568 mg)	

Mineral/vitamin mix – Dog and cat servings are the same, but formulas are different

Cups fed	Dog	Cat
¼ c	1/32 t	1/32 t
½ c	1/16 t	1/16 t
1 c	⅛ t	⅛ t
2 c	¼ t	¼ t
3 c	⅜ t	⅜ t
4 c	½ t	½ t
5 c	½ t +	
6 c	¾ t	
7 c	¾ t +	
8 c	1 t	

Turkey fatty acid supplement – amounts differ for turkey and chicken: use both oils!

Cups fed	Flax Oil	Krill Oil
¼ c	⅛ t	35 mg
½ c	¼ t	75 mg
1 c	½ t	125 mg
2 c	1 t	250 mg
3 c	1 ½ t	375 mg
4 c	2 t	500 mg
5 c	2 ½ t	625 mg
6 c	2 ¾ t	750 mg
7 c	1 T	1000 mg
8 c	3 ½ t	1125 mg

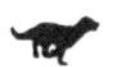

An egg meal – Feed the equivalent of 1 egg meal a week

AN EGG MEAL = Eggs + Pumpkin + Mineral/Vitamin Mix

If it's more convenient or tasty for your pet, you can include the eggs with other meals, keeping the proportions of "meat" and "veggies" the same. Reduce the meat mix by 4 Tablespoons per egg added. The addition or subtraction of the pumpkin makes little difference overall, but pumpkin is an easy addition to any meal and keeps well refrigerated.

Eggs may be fed lightly cooked or raw. If you are concerned that raw egg whites may interfere with biotin absorption, cook the eggs slightly so that whites are cooked. We don't think it's necessary. However, the people and dog "egg fest" is very popular with dogs, who love it when everybody eats together. Cats may enjoy it, too. Eggs are best cooked over easy, or soft cooked. When the yolk stays uncooked and unbroken, all the fragile fatty acids are preserved. If you are concerned about bacteria, cooking eggs will kill possible bacteria. In this case, cook the yolk until it is solid. Eggs are best eaten as soon as they are cooked.

You can easily multiply this recipe up or scale it down. You want to end up with the volume of food your pet eats for a meal. For example, if your dog eats a cup of food per meal, that cup of egg food contains 4 eggs. That's how many eggs are needed per week to provide the nutrients that eggs add to this program.

If you choose to add the eggs to other meals, calculate how many eggs per week are needed for your dog or cat and spread them over the week. Adjust down an equal amount on the meat mix part of the meal if you choose to spread your eggs out over the course of a week so you don't add too many calories or unbalance other nutrients.

No oil or calcium supplements are needed for this meal. We've included the "bone" requirement elsewhere in the rotation for the week. Fatty acid adjustment is not needed. Add mineral mix if you are feeding a whole meal of eggs.

Prepare the eggs as you wish, add the pumpkin and mineral supplement.

Add enzymes, glandular, probiotics and other supplements at mealtime as well, using product guidelines.

Dog egg meal – Feed 1 egg meal a week

May be fed as part of other meals.

Cups fed	Eggs (high omega-3)	Pumpkin
½ c food	2 large eggs	2 T pumpkin
1 c food	4 large eggs	¼ c pumpkin
2 c food	7 large eggs	½ c pumpkin
3 c food	10 large eggs	¾ c pumpkin
4 c food	14 large eggs	1 c pumpkin

Cat egg meal – Feed 1 egg meal a week

May be fed as part of other meals.

Cups fed	Eggs (high omega-3)	Pumpkin
½ c food	2 large eggs	1 T pumpkin
1 c food	4 large eggs	2 T pumpkin
2 c food	8 large eggs	2 oz pumpkin

Mineral/vitamin mix – Dog and cat servings are the same, but formulas are different

Use this table if you feed your pet a whole meal of eggs (eggs and pumpkin mixed).

Cups fed	Dog	Cat
¼ c	1/32 t	1/32 t
½ c	1/16 t	1/16 t
1 c	⅛ t	⅛ t
2 c	¼ t	¼ t
3 c	⅜ t	⅜ t
4 c	½ t	½ t
5 c	½ t +	
6 c	¾ t	
7 c	¾ t +	
8 c	1 t	

A sardine meal – Feed the equivalent of 1 sardine meal a week

A SARDINE MEAL = Sardines + Veggie Puree + Mineral/Vitamin Mix

Sardines are very convenient. Open the can and serve! There are no bone additions to this meal because the bone is already in the fish. As with eggs, if you want to include sardines as part of other meals that's perfectly fine.

If you've never fed your dog or cat sardines, start slowly. This is a fat-rich, calorie-dense meal. Start by adding one or two sardines to your dog's food, or a piece of a sardine for a cat, or give them as treats. If all goes well, with no digestive upsets, proceed to whole meals.

For animals who have any history of problems with fat, spreading out sardines in other meals is a good plan. This may also be a good idea for cats with addictive personalities who could decide to eat only sardines.

"Fish breath" is part of a sardine meal, so there's something to be said for having it a meal instead of a daily occurrence, but if spreading out the fish during a week works for you, feel free to do that.

Adjust down an equal amount on the meat mix part of the meal if you choose to spread your fish out over the course of a week so you don't add too many calories or unbalance other nutrients. The weekly amount of sardines needed equals the amount per meal on the chart opposite. For example, if your dog eats 2 cups of food per meal, spread 3 ½ cans of sardines over a week (and eat the other ½ can yourself). Add some pumpkin and greens to your overall veggie balance if you spread out the sardines, keeping meat mix and veggie puree balance the same, but it will not make a big difference to most animals if you don't.

Like the egg meal, this meal is best made and fed. There's no benefit in opening a bunch of cans and then freezing the contents! You may substitute frozen sardines or frozen ground sardines (made by raw pet food companies). **Buy sardines in water.** Sardines packed in oil can be drained, but the oils used are not the best quality and many calories are added to a meal even if the oil is drained. The recipe is computed on drained weight, about a pound of sardines for the dog meal, but you can include the water.

If you're serving a sardine meal, mix the ingredients at right, add minerals and serve. Add enzymes, glandular, probiotics and other supplements at mealtime as well, using product guidelines.

Dog sardine meal – Feed 1 sardine meal a week

May be fed as part of other meals. Based on cans with drained weight of 95 grams.

Cups fed	Sardines	Pumpkin	Pureed greens (anything that has color!)
½ c	1 can	1 ½ T pumpkin	2 t pureed greens
1 c	2 cans	3 T pumpkin	1 T pureed greens
2 c	3 ½ cans	¼ c pumpkin	2 T pureed greens
3 c	5 ½ cans	½ c pumpkin	¼ c pureed greens
4 c	7 cans	½ c pumpkin	¼ c + pureed greens

Cat sardine meal – Feed 1 sardine meal a week

May be fed as part of other meals.

Cups fed	Sardines	Pumpkin	Pureed greens (anything that has color!)
½ c	1 can	1 T+ pumpkin	2 t pureed greens
1 c	2 cans	2 T pumpkin	1 t pureed greens
2 c	4 ¼ cans	3 T pumpkin	1 T pureed greens

Mineral/vitamin mix – Dog and cat servings are the same, but formulas are different

Cups fed	Dog	Cat
¼ c	1/32 t	1/32 t
½ c	1/16 t	1/16 t
1 c	⅛ t	⅛ t
2 c	¼ t	¼ t
3 c	⅜ t	⅜ t
4 c	½ t	½ t
5 c	½ t +	
6 c	¾ t	
7 c	¾ t +	
8 c	1 t	

Small recipe boneless chicken or turkey

Feed 5 chicken meals *and* two turkey meals a week

A POULTRY MEAL = Meat Mix + Veggie Puree + Bone Supplement + Mineral/Vitamin Mix + Krill + Flax

• Poultry mix for dogs or cats

12 oz (1 ½ c) lean chicken or turkey thighs or breasts with some skin (use some gizzards if available)

3 oz (⅓ c +) chicken or turkey heart (or freeze dried equivalent)

1 oz (2 T) chicken or turkey liver (or freeze dried equivalent)

Grind or chop meat ingredients and mix well.

• Veggie puree suggestions for small recipes

Veggie puree for small recipes may be made in quantities that will keep for two or three days, but don't make more than this unless you plan to freeze to prevent loss of nutrients. For longer storage, freeze. The combinations below are just examples. Use what you have available and strive to include lots of color and variety.

ONE	TWO	THREE
8 oz (1 c) broccoli	8 oz (1 c) cooked sweet potato, no skin	8 oz (1 c) zucchini
4 oz (½ c) celery	1 oz (2 T) papaya	2 oz (¼ c) chard
2 oz (¼ c) blueberries	2 oz (¼ c) romaine	3 oz (⅓ c) red or orange pepper
2 oz (¼ c) watermelon	2 oz (¼ c) apple	1 oz (2 T) raspberries

Wash produce and drain. Skin sweet potato if using. Chop roughly and puree in batches your blender or food processor can handle, with a little water as needed.

These amounts are only for a day or two. The dog recipe makes a day's worth of food for a medium size dog, and the cat recipe perhaps 3 days. Add calcium supplement, mineral/ vitamin mix and oils to the whole recipe.

- **Combine meat and veggie puree and add supplements to entire poultry mix**

FOR DOGS

Combine meat mix with veggie puree, add supplements below and blend well.

2 g	(2142 mg) calcium (bone supplement that supplies specified amount of calcium)
5.4 oz	(scant ¾ c) veggie puree (suggestions on previous page)
1 t	flax oil for turkey OR ½ t flax oil for chicken
250 mg	krill oil
¼ t	mineral/vitamin mix

FOR CATS

Combine meat mix with veggie puree, add supplements below and blend well.

1.6 g	(1600 mg) calcium (bone supplement that supplies specified amount of calcium)
2.7 oz	(scant ⅓ c) veggie puree (suggestions on previous page)
1 t	flax oil for turkey OR ½ t flax oil for chicken
250 mg	krill oil
¼ t	mineral/vitamin mix

Add enzymes, glandular, probiotics and other supplements at mealtimes, using product guidelines.

Small recipe boneless beef – Feed 5 beef meals a week

A BEEF MEAL = Meat Mix + Veggie Puree + Bone Supplement + Mineral/Vitamin Mix + Krill + Hemp

• Beef mix for dogs or cats

12 oz (1 ½ c) lean beef

3 oz (1/3 c +) beef heart

1 oz (2 T) beef liver

Grind or chop meat ingredients and mix well.

• Veggie puree suggestions for small recipes

Veggie puree for small recipes may be made in quantities that will keep for two or three days, but don't make more than this unless you plan to freeze to prevent loss of nutrients. For longer storage, freeze. The combinations below are just examples. Use what you have available and strive to include lots of color and variety.

ONE	TWO	THREE
8 oz (1 c) broccoli	8 oz (1 c) cooked sweet potato, no skin	8 oz (1 c) zucchini
4 oz (½ c) celery	1 oz (2 T) papaya	2 oz (¼ c) chard
2 oz (¼ c) blueberries	2 oz (¼ c) romaine	3 oz (1/3 c) red or orange pepper
2 oz (¼ c) watermelon	2 oz (¼ c) apple	1 oz (2 T) raspberries
		2 oz (¼ c) cantaloupe

Wash produce and drain. Skin sweet potato. Chop roughly and puree in batches your blender or food processor can handle, with a little water as needed.

These amounts are only for a day or two. The dog recipe makes a day's worth of food for a medium size dog, and the cat recipe perhaps 2 or 3 days. Add calcium supplement, mineral/ vitamin mix and oils to the whole recipe.

- **Combine meat and veggie puree and add supplements to entire beef mix**

FOR DOGS

Combine meat mix with veggie puree, add supplements below and blend well.

2 g	(2142 mg) calcium (bone supplement that supplies specified amount of calcium)
5.7 oz	(scant ¾ c) veggie puree (suggestions previous page)
1 t	hemp oil
250 mg	krill oil
¼ t	mineral/vitamin mix

FOR CATS

Combine meat mix with veggie puree, add supplements below and blend well.

1.6 g	(1600 mg) calcium (bone supplement that supplies specified amount of calcium)
2.7 oz	(1/3 c) veggie puree (suggestions previous page)
1 t	hemp
250 mg	krill oil
¼ t	mineral/vitamin mix

Add enzymes, glandular, probiotics and other supplements at mealtime as well, using product guidelines.

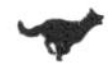

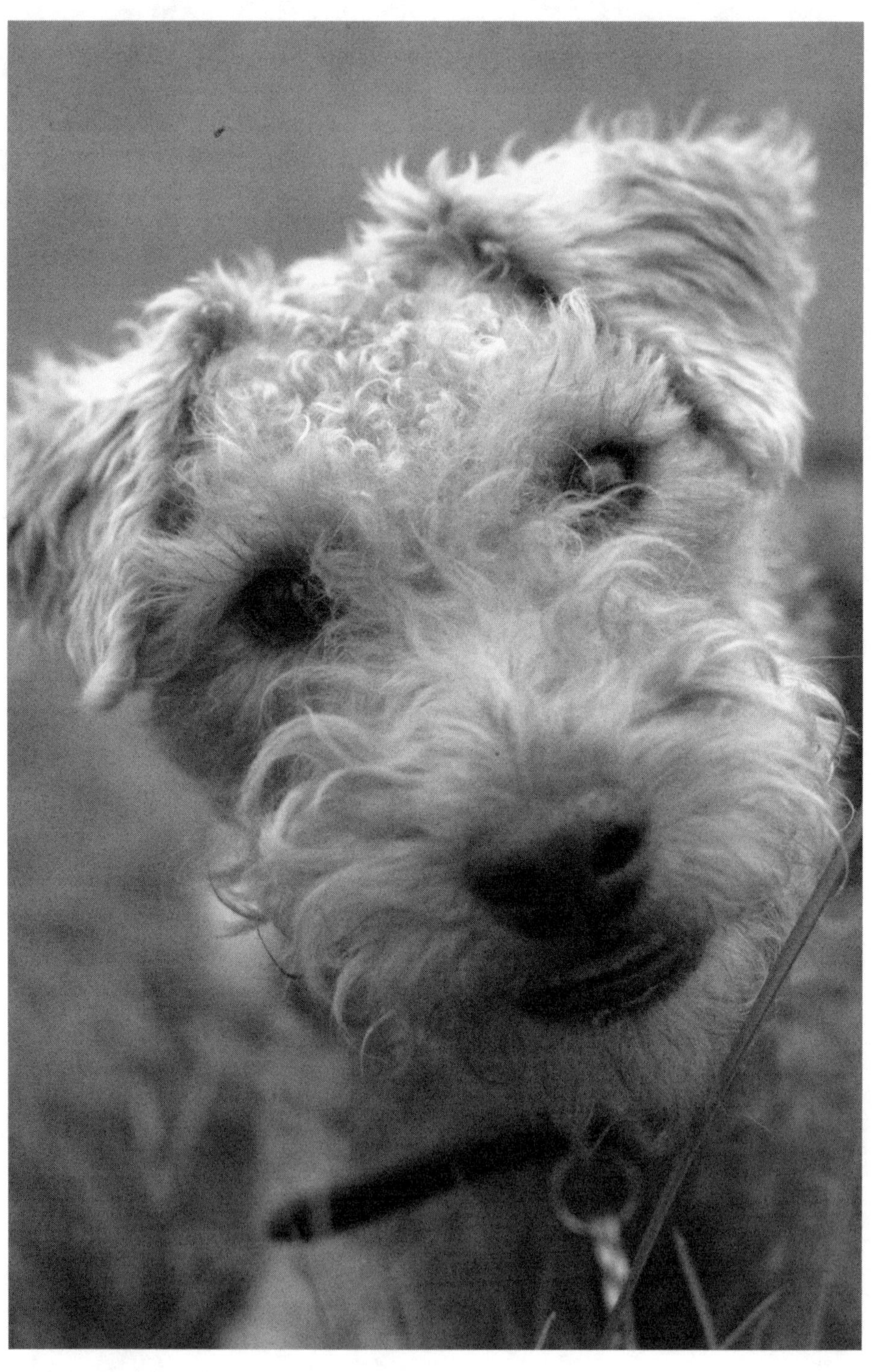

RECIPES WITH GROUND BONE AND ORGANS

The poultry recipes that follow are a "next step," for those who wish to include fresh bone in their dog or cat food. The proportions give you the proper ratio of bone to meat. Do not cook recipes with whole or ground bone. If you make chicken food with bone, a small grinder will do. If you make turkey food, you need a large grinder to handle the larger bones. You don't see a beef recipe because beef bones are too hard to grind in a home grinder of any sort. You can feed some whole, raw beef bones but it's hard to estimate proportions. We suggest that you stick to the beef recipe with bone meal to ensure that you have the right balance and provide your dog with the occasional recreational knuckle bone, or your cat with a chicken neck, if it's appropriate for your animal. Check with your holistic veterinarian about proper bite (tooth alignment) and general health.

A bone supplement is not included in these recipes. Necks provide bone. Because a cat's dietary bone requirement is different than that of a dog, the proportions in the recipes are also different. Veggie purees are included and can be added to your meat mix when you make it, or added in appropriate amounts when you feed your pet.

We prefer for this simple program that you just grind your food with bone, but you may choose to use our proportions to feed whole turkey and chicken necks to your animals (do not feed whole turkey necks to cats). If you choose to keep necks whole, make sure that you include the proper amount of meat and organs specified in the rest of the recipe. Refer to the "meat with bone" discussion in the meat section about adding raw bone to your animal's diet, and to our DVD, *Fast Fresh Functional Food for Furry Friends* for an in-depth discussion. Don't feed whole meals of chicken necks or other bony parts!

Whole birds also give you a good balance of bone to meat. Disjointing chickens for grinding is a large, messy project. Turkeys, being bigger, require the use of more muscle power and a large cleaver to get pieces small enough to fit in the (large) grinder. Give them a try if you have the equipment and you're inclined. You can make food very cheaply this way. If you grind whole birds, add together the weight of the meat and neck amounts in each recipe and use that amount of ground-up bird for the meat portion of the meat mix recipe — you still add the organs.

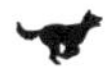

Chicken with bone and organs – do not cook this mix!

Feed 5 chicken meals a week

A CHICKEN WITH BONE MEAL = Meat Mix + Veggie Puree + Mineral/Vitamin Mix + Krill + Flax

• Meat Mix

Dogs

4.5# (9 c ground) chicken necks, skinless

4.5# (9 c ground) boneless chicken breast, thigh (and gizzards too)

1# (2 c ground) chicken heart (or freeze dried equivalent)

½# (1 c ground) chicken liver

Cats

2.5# (5 c ground) chicken necks, skinless

6.5# (7 c ground) boneless chicken breast, thigh (and gizzards too)

1# (2 c ground) chicken heart (or freeze dried equivalent)

½ # (1 c ground) chicken liver

Grind necks, and chop or grind other ingredients. Mix well.

• Veggie and fruit puree for chicken with bone

For dogs

1# (2 c) carrots

1# (2 c) Chinese cabbage

1# (2 c) red or yellow peppers

8 oz (1 c) cantaloupe

For cats

8 oz (1 c) carrots

8 oz (1 c) Chinese cabbage

8 oz (1 c) red or yellow peppers

4 oz (½ c) cantaloupe

Wash produce and drain. Chop roughly and puree in batches your blender or food processor can handle, with a little water as needed.

• Combine meat mix with veggie puree

There are two ways to combine meat mix with veggie puree.

1. Combine the entire meat mix recipe with the entire veggie puree recipe for your species. Proportions of meat and veggies will be correct.
2. Freeze veggie puree and meat mix separately and mix at time of feeding.

Below are proportions for combining meat and veggies after thawing.

Meat mix to veggie puree proportions for cats and dogs

DOGS 3 parts meat mix to 1 part veggies = 3 c meat mix + 1 c veggies
CATS 7 parts meat mix to 1 part veggies = 7/8 c meat mix + 1/8 c veggies

Freeze in convenient amounts to use within a day or two after thawing.

• Add supplements at mealtimes

Add mineral/vitamin mix and both oils at mealtimes, using the tables below. Amounts given are for meat mix with veggie puree added. Add enzymes, glandular, probiotics and other supplements at mealtimes as well, using product guidelines.

There is no bone supplement table for this recipe. The bone is included in the recipe.

It's possible to adapt these "with bone" recipes for feeding whole necks, but beyond the capacity of this little book to discuss adequately. You'll find a couple of paragraphs on this topic in the "meat" section. Our DVD, *Fast Functional Food for Furry Friends*, discusses this topic in depth. If you're interested in taking this step, please consult our DVD!

Mineral/vitamin supplement

Cups fed	Dog	Cat
¼ c	1/32 t	1/32 t
½ c	1/16 t	1/16 t
1 c	1/8 t	1/8 t
2 c	¼ t	¼ t
3 c	3/8 t	3/8 t
4 c	½ t	½ t
5 c	½ t +	
6 c	¾ t	
7 c	¾ t +	
8 c	1 t	

Fatty acid supplements for chicken: amounts are different for chicken and turkey

Cups fed	Flax Oil	Krill Oil
¼ c	4 drops	35 mg
½ c	1/8 t	75 mg
1 c	¼ t	125 mg
2 c	½ t	250 mg
3 c	1 t	375 mg
4 c	1 ½ t	500 mg
5 c	1 ¾ t	625 mg
6 c	2 t	750 mg
7 c	2 ½ t	1000 mg
8 c	2 ¾ t	1125 mg

Turkey with bone and organs – do not cook this mix!

Feed 5 chicken meals a week

A TURKEY WITH BONE MEAL = Meat Mix + Veggie Puree + Mineral/Vitamin Mix + Krill + Flax

• Meat Mix

Dogs

4.5#	(9 c ground) turkey necks, skinless
4.5#	(9 c ground) turkey breast, boneless thigh (and gizzards too)
1#	(2 c ground) turkey heart (or freeze dried equivalent)
½#	(1 c ground) turkey liver (or freeze dried equivalent)

Cats

2.5#	(5 c ground) turkey necks, skinless – always grind for cats!
6.5#	(7 c ground) turkey breast, boneless thigh (and gizzards too)
1#	(2 c ground) turkey heart (or freeze dried equivalent)
½#	(1 c ground) turkey liver (or freeze dried equivalent)

Grind necks, and chop or grind other ingredients. Mix well.

• Veggie and fruit puree for turkey

For dogs		For cats	
1 ½#	(3 c) zucchini	12 oz	(1½ c) zucchini
7 oz	(7/8 c) apple	3 ½ oz	(scant ½ c) apple
1 ½#	(3 c) cooked sweet potato	10 oz	(¾ c) cooked sweet potato
4 oz	(½ c) papaya	2 oz	(¼ c) papaya

Bake sweet potatoes and remove from skin. Discard skin. Starchy vegetables are better digested if they are cooked. Wash produce and drain. Chop roughly and puree in batches your blender or food processor can handle, with a little water as needed.

• Combine meat mix with veggie puree

There are two ways to combine meat mix with veggie puree.

1. Combine the entire meat mix recipe with the entire veggie puree recipe for your species. Proportions of meat and veggies will be correct.
2. Freeze veggie puree and meat mix separately and mix at time of feeding.

Below are proportions for combining meat and veggies after thawing.

Meat mix to veggie puree proportions for cats and dogs

DOGS 3 parts meat mix to 1 part veggies = 3 c meat mix + 1 c veggies
CATS 7 parts meat mix to 1 part veggies = 7/8 c meat mix + 1/8 c veggies

Freeze in convenient amounts to use within a day or two after thawing.

• Add supplements at mealtimes

Add mineral/vitamin mix and both oils at mealtimes, using the tables below. Amounts given are for meat mix with veggie puree added. Add enzymes, glandular, probiotics and other supplements at mealtimes as well, using product guidelines.

There is no bone supplement table for this recipe. The bone is included in the recipe.

It's possible to adapt these "with bone" recipes for feeding whole necks, but beyond the capacity of this little book to discuss adequately. You'll find a couple of paragraphs on this topic in the "meat" section. Our DVD, *Fast Functional Food for Furry Friends*, discusses this topic in depth. If you're interested in taking this step, please consult our DVD!

Mineral/vitamin supplement

Cups fed	Dog	Cat
¼ c	1/32 t	1/32 t
½ c	1/16 t	1/16 t
1 c	⅛ t	⅛ t
2 c	¼ t	¼ t
3 c	⅜ t	⅜ t
4 c	½ t	½ t
5 c	½ t +	
6 c	¾ t	
7 c	¾ t +	
8 c	1 t	

Fatty acid supplements for turkey: use both oils!

Cups fed	Flax Oil	Krill Oil
¼ c	4 drops	35 mg
½ c	⅛ t	75 mg
1 c	½ t	125 mg
2 c	1 t	250 mg
3 c	1 ½ t	375 mg
4 c	1 ¾ t	500 mg
5 c	2 t	625 mg
6 c	2 ½ t	750 mg
7 c	1 T	1000 mg
8 c	3 ½ t	1125 mg

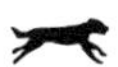

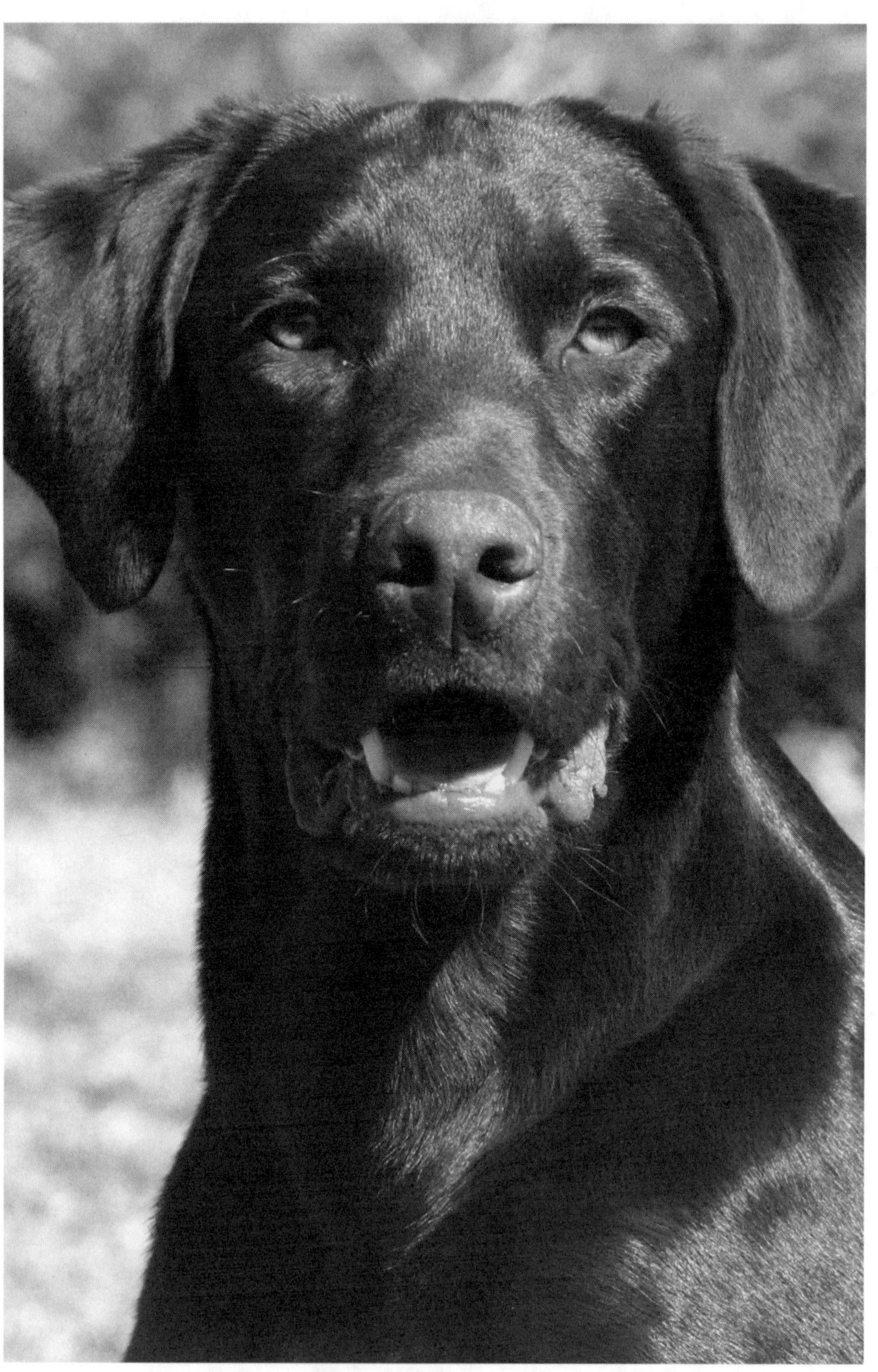

HOW MUCH DO I FEED MY ANIMALS?

It seems that there should be an easy way to figure out how much food to feed your pet, but there's not. You need to know your pet and you need to develop some skill in evaluating your pet's condition. There are good charts to help you evaluate whether your dog or cat is thin or fat, but breed type, age and other factors make it more complicated than just looking at a chart.

Some dogs are stocky and muscular, with heavy bones. Even thin, they weigh more than lightly boned and muscled dogs of the same general size. A Rottweiler and a Saluki might be the same height, but that's about where the similarities end! Different breeds and breed types have different metabolisms. Cat breeds and body types display the same differences, from the slender and elongated to the stocky and muscular.

Young and old animals may eat different amounts. When your 50 pound Labrador Retriever is six months old, for example, she may eat four pounds of food a day. When she is a mature, active three year old, she might be down to two pounds per day. As an old girl, maybe only one pound.

If the Labrador above were a Basset Hound of equal weight, he would probably eat less than this. Bassets tend to need less food than many other breeds. A German Shorthair Pointer may burn a lot of food for years, or forever. Pointers can use a lot of calories just keeping warm! Some dogs are built for cold weather and some for hot. Seasonal differences affect how much food your dog needs.

Small dogs burn more food for their size than big dogs and they mature much earlier. Girl dogs tend to start putting on weight at puberty, unlike boy dogs (sound familiar, humans?). The effects of spaying and neutering on metabolism are hotly debated and we won't try to cover that topic here, but in general most pets need fewer calories after de-sexing. Clearly, there are many variables and every cat and dog is different.

Puppies and kittens may eat twice as much as adults. Learn the growth habits of your breed and your pet's family when it's possible so you'll have an idea what to expect. For example, one line of Golden Retrievers may be slowing down and maturing at 18 months, while another line is still skinny and adolescent at three years. Those with no way to obtain family history must rely on observation, but there is much to be learned from body type. If your dog looks like a German Shepherd, he may grow like a German Shepherd. If he's a ten pound curly mixed-breed, he might grow up fast, like a poodle.

Overweight animals should not lose weight too rapidly. Start out feeding them for slightly under their current weight and adjust so that they lose no more than 1 – 2% of their body weight per month. For example, your Labrador weighs 80 pounds. You're not sure, but you think she should weigh 65 pounds. Figure out how much food she should eat for 75 pounds and feed her that for a week or two. If no weight loss occurs, reduce the amount. Keep reducing as you go. At 75 pounds, feed her for 70 pounds. If your dog is obese, enlist assistance from your veterinarian to monitor her health during weight loss and use 1-2% of body weight per month as a guide.

At the other end of the scale, we see dogs that are underweight. They are often performance dogs whose people want them to be as healthy as possible and to them, this means thin. This often happens, too, when dogs are switched to fresh food and start out a bit chubby. Owners get very enthusiastic about their pet's new waistline and just keep going. Ribs and spines should not stick out unless your breed is built that way. Muscular breeds should have muscle. Fat is needed in the body for many functional reasons. Dogs that are too thin cannot even build the proper amount of muscle for their body structure. This is an unhealthy state.

Cats are often very resistant when it comes to diet change. Make sure your cat is transitioning acceptably. Cats must eat daily or they can have terrible metabolic problems. Obese cats may do best being weaned off dry food and onto canned food, then off canned food onto homemade cooked food, then onto homemade raw food. Obese cats must be dieted very slowly and with the help and supervision of a veterinarian.

If you are switching your overweight dog or cat from dry food to fresh food, it's common to see a significant weight loss in the first week. This is usually the result of the body letting go of water retained due to the inflammatory effects of grain-based food. It's quite impressive, but future weight loss should take place more gradually.

Your food scale will help you keep track of how much you're really feeding. If you always feed your dog one pound of food a day and now he's getting fat or thin, you need to know why, and you need to be sure you know how much you're really giving him.

Is this a seasonal thing? He needs less in the summer, more in the winter, or the reverse? If you're sure you're giving him the same amount, you can look at exercise, activity and other factors in making sure that all is well.

If he's losing weight on the same amount of food, there might be trouble brewing — or you might have changed the composition of the food, or conditions have changed. For example, we know one dog who lost several pounds from his 20 pound body when his owner took a three month break from agility training — less exercise for the dog, but no training treats! His owner was afraid he was ill, but when his food level was adjusted, he was fine. On the other hand, weight loss can point to many different health problems, including parasites. Don't ignore unexpected weight loss.

The charts for feeding amounts are given in cups for general guidelines. We show you a range of food amounts that may be appropriate for your pet and traditional kitchen measurements you can use to make sense of it all.

The best way to find out what's right for your pet is to start somewhere in the middle range and see how it goes. Active and young animals start toward the top of the range, and older or chubby animals in the middle. Evaluate you pet's condition frequently! Too much food may cause digestive upset or weight gain. Too little and your dog may be so thin that his body is unable to maintain vital functions.

Directions are based on the calorie count of our recipes. The recipes have been analyzed and compared to the ancestral diet, the requirements of the organization that regulates pet food (AAFCO), and the recommendations of the National Research Council, to make sure they supply needed nutrients. The high end of recommendations in the chart is usually the "official" caloric range. Fresh food veterans agree that animals often maintain weight and condition on ⅓ fewer calories than those recommendations. We've included the entire range of recommendations.

There really are no fast, easy answers. Only experience will show you what's right for your animal.

For dogs, recipes average 35 calories per ounce, 560 calories per pound. The cat recipes average 39 calories per ounce, 624 calories per pound. The difference is in the lower veggie content of the cat recipe.

Don't get too attached to the categories on following pages. Your individual dog may stay in the food range of a "young/working" dog all his life. Or, he may graduate to the "older/inactive" category when he's two, even though he's pretty active. The amounts are given as a guideline. Each animal is different. "Official" calorie recommendations are based on results with animals eating dry food. In our experience, real food is quite different.

The amount of food that a young, active dog can eat may seem immense. Dry food packs a lot of calories into a cup. Real food, which has all the water still in it, often has less than half the calories of dry food. You'll get used to the volume of real food, but the actual number of calories your dog consumes is likely to be less than what's recommended — even though it may seem like a lot of food!

At the other end of the spectrum, our "mature," healthy dogs usually eat at the low end of the "inactive" category, unless they are very active. If you calculated the calorie count, it wouldn't seem likely given the charts, but that's our real life experience. Don't assume it will be your experience, but be aware that it's not unusual.

Suggested range of amounts to feed per day

Divide amount by number of meals fed. Totals are for food with veggies.

CAT	Kitten 3-5 months	Adult Active	Adult Moderately Active	Adult Older/Inactive
1#	⅓ c			
2#	¾ c			
3#	½ – 1 c			
4#	¾ – 1 ⅓ c	Scant ½ c	⅓ c	¼ c plus
5#		½ c plus	½ c	⅓ c plus
7#		¾ c	Scant ¾ c	½ c
9#		1 c	Scant 1 c	¾ c
11#		1 ¼ c	1 c plus	Scant 1 c
13#		1 ½ c	1 ¼ c	1 c
15#		1 ¾ c	1 ½ c	1 ¼ c

Few 15-17 pound cats are at their proper weight! Help your cat lose extra ounces with veterinary supervision that considers general health and condition, so they lose at a rate that's safe.

DOG	Puppies	Young/ working	Active Adult	Adult Older/Inactive
5#	1 ¾ c	1 c	¾ c	⅓ c
10#	2 ¾ c	2 c	1 ¼ c	1 c
20#	4 – 5 c	2 ¾ – 3 ½ c	1¾ – 2 c	1 ¼ – 1 ¾ c
30#	5 ¾ – 7 c	4 – 4 ½ c	2 ⅓ – 2 ¾ c	1 ¾ – 2 ⅓ c
40#*	6 – 6 ½ c	5 ¼ – 5 ¾ c	3 – 3 ½ c	2 ¼ – 2 ¾ c
50#	7 – 7 ⅔ c	6 ⅓ – 6 ⅞ c	3 ¾ – 4 c	2 ¾ – 3 ½ c
60#	8 ¼ – 8 ¾ c	7 ⅓ – 8 ¼ c	4 ⅓ – 4 ⅔ c	3 – 4 c
70#	9 ⅓ – 10 c	8 ⅓ – 8 ¼ c	5 – 5 ¼ c	3 ⅔ – 4 ½ c
80 #	10 ⅓ – 11 c	9 ¼ – 9 ¾ c	5 ½ – 5 ¾ c	4 – 5 c
90#	12 – 13 c	10 – 10 ⅓ c	6 – 6 ¼	4 ⅓ – 5 ½ c

* We assumed in the puppy column above that few puppies over 40 pounds would be at less than 50% of their adult weight. So, for puppies 40 pounds and over, we've given you amounts for pups from 50 – 80% of their adult weight. For puppies 5 – 30 pounds, amounts are for pups less than 50% of body weight.

SUCCESSFUL SWITCHING

Change your pet over to real food in a way that makes sense to you. It might take a while for you to get comfortable with the whole idea and that's fine. However, your animal's body is probably ready for a new concept in food today and you'll be a hero when you start handing out real food. The total switch can often be accomplished within a week.

Start by feeding your dog or cat a little bit of fresh food and see how he does with it. If all is well, keep adding a little bit, but start taking out some of his old food. If things are going well, you can usually remove the old food within a few days. Another option is to add the new food as a mid-day snack, to see how he handles it.

If you need to keep feeding some dry food, figure out the appropriate daily amount of fresh food and the daily amount of dry food and use fractions of that daily ration to base your plan on. For example, Rusty eats a cup of dry food a day. You calculate that he would eat a pound of fresh food a day. So, feed him half of his dry food ration (half a cup) in the morning. Moisten the dry food with warm water before feeding. Rehydrating food makes it easier to digest. In the evening, feed him a half-pound of fresh food (half his daily fresh food ration). Feeding dry food in the morning allows your pet to burn off the carbohydrates in the grain-based dry food during the day. It's best to keep the dry food separate from the fresh, uncooked food. This is just one example. Each individual might be treated differently.

Calculate fresh and dry food separately. Dry food and fresh or canned food have very different calorie counts due to the water in wet foods and the absence of water in dry foods. One cup of dry food has many more calories than one cup of fresh or frozen food, which still contains all the natural water. If you're using commercial foods, know the calorie count per pound or ounce so that you can be accurate.

Take this difference into consideration, or you might find yourself seriously underfeeding your dog or cat in the process of switching. We have talked to many people who thought that fresh food was bad for their dog because he lost so much weight. In fact, they were still feeding the one cup a day that was the dog's dry food ration. When the amount was adjusted and he was fed more, he thrived.

If your pet has loose stools, wait until the stool is firm to continue the transition. If loose stools continue, consult your holistic veterinarian.

You may feed your pet once a day or twice a day. Puppies and kittens are fed frequently as babies and less frequently as they mature. Old animals sometimes do better with frequent feedings, as do ill and recovering animals. Otherwise, observe your pet and see what plan you think works best.

Cats frequently have strong opinions about diet changes. It sounds simple to just switch your cat's food—after all, meat tastes better than dry food! Your cat may disagree. Dry foods are designed to be tasty, and many cats are addicted to the salt, fat and sugar included. Often, cats are not open to the idea of variety, especially if they have only been fed one food (as we have been advised by pet food companies for decades). Creativity and patience may be needed to switch your cat.

It may sound odd, but it's important to not care too much about the end result (both in how you behave and how you think and feel about this). Even though you might know that this is the absolute best thing for your cat, if you make too big a thing of it in your mind or your actions you may set off resistance in your cat. Cats are good at sensing tension. This is sometimes the case with dogs too, but dogs usually say, "Right! Food!" Cats, on the other hand, often say, "You must be joking!"

Cats will starve themselves. They are not good candidates for the "tough love" approach. Some very serious conditions can occur if cats do not eat for an extended period, especially if cats are overweight. A slow switch will prevent problems. That said, a healthy animal that has an opportunity to become a bit hungry will make the switch more easily. This is one reason that we strongly recommend that you pick up the dry food dish and move immediately to meals at times that are appropriate for your cat. Check with your veterinarian about what's safe for your cat.

Feed multiple cats separately.

Establish regular feeding times and put food away in between meals. For many reasons, it's best for the body not to have food available all the time. If you have dogs, you know what to do with leftovers!

Consider dry food to be a snack only, not left out all the time — use a few pieces as a treat. This is the equivalent of "kitty junk food," part of the transition — eventually you are headed toward no dry food at all. **It's our experience that you must put away the "free feed" bowl in order to have success.**

Consider weaning dry food junkies onto canned food first, then mix small amounts (very small amounts!) of homemade food into canned food.

Offer bits of fresh food that you are eating. They may refuse, but one day… they won't. Your goal is to get your cat to consider things as food other than dry, crunchy items.

Cat whiskers are very sensitive. If food is served in a bowl that interferes with whiskers, it could be enough to keep the cat from considering the food. A flat dish works well.

Trickery sometimes works with cats. Put the food on YOUR plate, or hide it in a location cats know to be forbidden… creativity helps!

Cats generally prefer their food between room temperature and body temperature. Warming food releases the flavors and fragrances. Cats choose food by smell. Wet food is a lot less fragrant than a dry food they have been eating. This is often the reason that the second half of a can of food is refused — the first time it was at room temperature.

Consider the personality of your cat during the switching process and when planning meals. We recommend one fish meal a week, but if your cat is the type to go on strike for fish, it might be better to spread that fish over the week.

If you're on your way to fresh food with your cat, but not there yet, additions for canned and dry diets can improve things a lot. Add a sardine for good fats, or use fish oil. One small sardine a day adds omega-3 fatty acids in their best form — whole food. If sardines don't appeal to you, you can use a fresh, well-preserved, omega-3 fish oil supplement with vitamin E.

Digestive enzymes and a glandular supplement are good additions to replace the parts of prey animals we normally don't feed, i.e. stomach and gut contents and the smaller glands. We use these as part of our fresh food program and they can be added to dry food and canned food as well, while you're working toward real food.

Live green food, which in the ancestral diet would be provided by grasses cats graze on, is important for good digestion. "Cat grass" which can be found in grocery and health food stores, is very popular with cats. You can grow your own from a kit, or simply grow some wheat or barley grass in a pot. This addition often takes the burden off the houseplants!

We think that the optimum diet for most cats is a **raw** meat-based or home cooked diet. The next best option is canned food. If you use canned food, your cat's diet will be fully hydrated. You will be much closer to providing him with optimum nutrition.

Canned foods that approximate the natural diet of a cat are the best choice. They're advertised as "grain-free." Make sure that you buy products that are "complete." In the "grain-free" products you may find products with plenty of sweet potatoes or potatoes or peas, making these foods starchier than we prefer. Check our website for a few current choices that we think have a good protein/fat/carbohydrate balance.

The worst choice for cats (and their kidneys) is dry food, even if the ingredients are impeccable. Cats need food that contains water.

A PRIMER OF COMMERCIAL FROZEN FOODS

In recent years, commercial fresh frozen diets and the stores and websites that specialize in healthier options for pets have multiplied and thrived. The products available have become more than an oddball special order item. Freezers filled with raw pet food are found even in big chain stores. These products can be very good and they can help you out when there's just not time to make food.

It's necessary to know your way around these foods. Store personnel are usually dedicated and concerned, but they don't always really know about the nutritional makeup of the foods. You need to know the calorie content, the amount of veggies and the fat/protein/carbohydrate amounts in order to compare.

There are two categories of commercial frozen foods. Complete diets are formulated to meet the AAFCO guidelines for all life stages. Component products are designed to allow you to put together your own diet.

The component products are very useful for providing more protein sources than are commonly available, and they often have frozen and freeze dried organ meats as part of their line. As long as you're aware that these are not complete diets, they can be great additions to your plan.

The complete products have a very wide range of nutrition profiles. This is where you can get into trouble if you're under-informed. The labels may say they are "complete" but the numbers may disagree.

To be close to the ancestral diet, label profiles must show about half as much fat as protein. For example, if a food is 12% protein, then it should be about 6% or 5% fat. Otherwise, many more fat calories are provided than protein. Since fat has more than twice as many calories as protein, it can easily displace protein in the diet, and you're quickly feeding your dog or cat a balance overwhelmingly on the fat side — often as much as 75-80% of the calories are fat. This is common in the diets that have almost no vegetables, but even in the higher veggie foods some varieties and brands may have high levels of fat. Fat is cheap and it makes the portion size smaller — and thus it can be cheaper to feed a higher fat food, but it's not the best choice unless your animals are active athletes who burn off the calories in healthy ways.

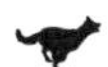

The inclusion of vegetables changes the profile considerably because they take up space. A low veggie 8 ounce patty might have 600 – 700 calories. 8 ounces of a higher veggie food might have 300 calories. Sales people may tell you that you're just paying for water in a higher veggie food. In fact, that water holds valuable nutrients.

These differences can make a scary change in an animal in a very short time. Fast and dangerous weight loss can occur, and just as swift weight gain, even if following the guidelines of the manufacturer or the store salesperson. A high fat diet fed to an animal whose digestive system is not in excellent shape (you may not know this) can lead to pancreatitis, which can be painful and even fatal. We can consult with you to help you choose an appropriate food.

Use caution when following feeding directions for commercial products. Recommendations are often made for very different products, which may not be immediately clear. For example, one brand sells both canned and raw frozen food, two products that seem similar. You might think that these could be substituted equally, but it's recommended that customers feed their pets twice as much canned food as raw food. In this case, the canned food has more water in it than the raw frozen food. The canned food has fewer calories per cup. If you fed your pet canned food according to the frozen directions, your dog would lose weight at an alarming rate. Read carefully and thoroughly! Directions are only a guideline.

We like to use the moderate products. For dogs, the ones that include 20-30% veggies and fruits by volume are the closest to our plan and to their evolutionary diet. For cats, the lower to very low veggie foods are appropriate, but they must also have appropriate fat content, a bit less than half the protein level given on the label. There are many choices, whether for foods to be shipped direct to your door or bought in a store. Check our website for resources for products we think are reliable and trouble free.

I READ ABOUT A GREAT SUPPLEMENT...

We're tempted by the health challenges of our companions to add supplements and herbs. Examine them well. In many cases, our animals have impaired digestion and supplements just won't be assimilated until digestive processes are restored and in balance.

"More" is not better

If your dog has "allergies," does it make sense to add an "immune booster" to an already over-reactive system? Probably not. It depends on how that substance acts in the body and on how the body processes it.

If your dog is not digesting food very well (like many dogs with "allergies"), an added substance won't be helpful and may irritate the system. If the liver is already overloaded, perhaps one more substance that is processed by the liver is not a good addition. Existing skin problems caused by an overloaded liver might flare up. Blood values may get worse.

If your dog is in pain and you're thinking of adding a supplement that promises a pain-free life, first remove any pro-inflammatory components in her diet. Grain-based dry food is the primary promoter of inflammation and pain in dogs and cats. You may not need that supplement at all if you eliminate the dietary source of inflammation. It makes better sense to remove a roadblock to health than to feed something that makes your pet feel bad and then give her a supplement (or drug) to take away the pain.

Even if an "expert" has recommended that you use a supplement, ask yourself the following questions:

- Do you understand how it works in the body? Will this substance put a burden on an overburdened body? Will it put other nutrients out of proportion? For example, mega-doses of Omega-3s may sound great — but in some cases they result in worsening of the symptom they were intended to help.
- Is it a whole food or an isolated, synthetic substance? Isolated nutrients don't provide the whole range of nutrients available from a food. In many cases, science has yet to uncover all the relationships, but more and more the conclusion of researchers is "eat whole food."

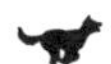

- Is it a combination of many "helpful" ingredients? Sensitive animals and those with impaired digestion are likely to be easily overloaded by "more."

The body takes time to heal. The immune system does not recover all at once. Digestion is complex. It includes not only processing nutrients, but also many critical immune functions. To fulfill all functions, everything has to be working. Be patient with the process.

FOOD FOR A LIFETIME

Maybe you started making food for your dog or cat because you want to maintain perfect health and you want to extend the good food program you follow to your pet. You learned about fresh food and decided that you have room in your life for the tasks involved in the process. If so, you're a hero.

Most of us began making food because we had a sick dog or cat. Fresh food was one of the main factors in returning our animals to health. We're grateful! But do we really have to keep doing this forever? Wouldn't our dog be fine if we fed him good dry food again? After all, the problems that brought us to making our own food are fixed, aren't they?

Perhaps you sometimes find yourself grinding your teeth as you look in the freezer and see that once again, the food is almost gone… time to do it all over again.

The basic questions are:

- Do I really have to do this?
- When can we go back to dry food?

The answers:

- Yes, you need to feed fresh food.
- No, you can never go back to dry food. Well, you can, but you sacrifice wellness.

The answer is simple. Real food is best.

The reason your pet is healthy now is that you feed him fresh food. If you had a sick animal, and he's better now, going back to dry food will bring back the problem — which was probably caused by nutrition originally. If you have been so successful that the entire problem is healed, give thanks.

Nutrition-induced conditions are often functional, not medical (though you may have spent thousands of dollars with veterinarians figuring out what's wrong). If you provide good food, fresh air, exercise and lots of love many conditions improve or heal themselves.

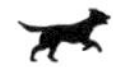

If you go back to the dry food routine that most of us started out with, your animal might be fine temporarily. But you should not be surprised to see old symptoms return eventually. Now that you know more than you did about how the body works you know that we can't always fix things that go wrong. Years later you could be faced with disease that progresses fast enough that diet change is no longer a simple solution.

If you just can't fit food preparation into your life, investigate commercial products. Maybe you can use them and make your own when you can.

There may be times when you must supplement with dry food for economic reasons, or just due to the fluctuations of life. Do the best you can and get back to healthier food as soon as it's workable in your life.

ENJOY YOURSELF AND YOUR ANIMALS!

When people start to learn about tools for healthier living for their animals, they find their lives changed in many ways.

It's possible to find a way to feed a meat-based, species-appropriate diet in almost any household, whether your tastes run to intensive or minimal preparation. The benefits of improving diet, however, extend far beyond the actual food.

Our lives are immeasurably enriched when we take the time to be involved in the process of living. We appreciate the miraculous world around us more and we become far better connected to our animals and each other.

We hope you find this to be true for yourself and all the animals who touch your life.

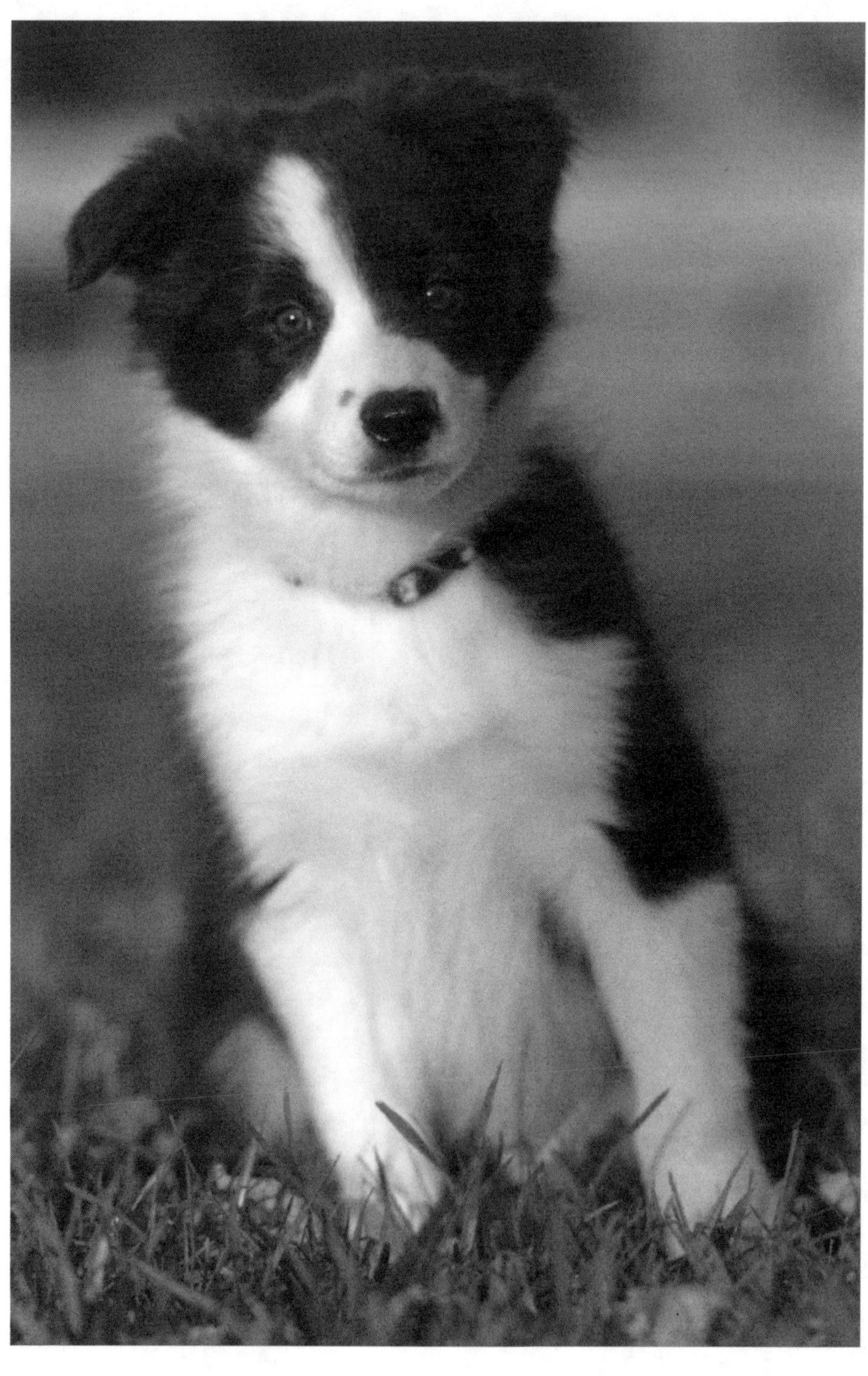

A PLEDGE

I am responsible for my health and wellbeing
and for that of the animals in my care.
I will become a knowledgeable advocate
for myself and my animals in all realms of life.

I understand that life, healing and health are always changing, requiring me to learn and evolve in order for me to become an effective advocate. I will not abdicate this responsibility to any person or doctor.

The health of my animals rests in my hands.

Beth Taylor, co-author of See Spot Live Longer, helps animal caretakers with food and lifestyle choices. Her interests include Traditional Chinese Medicine, massage and chiropractic. Beth lectures frequently on proactive health care and pet food topics for dog clubs, veterinary clinics and any group of interested individuals, and teaches observation and evaluation skills, and various massage techniques to small groups. Karen Becker is a veterinarian, animal acupuncturist and homeopath practicing in Illinois. Natural Pet Animal Hospital focuses on integrative pet care for dogs, cats, birds and exotic animals. She also runs Covenant Wildlife Rehabilitation, a non-profit facility that cares for injured and orphaned Chicago area wildlife. Together, for the past ten years, they have been producing seminars, DVDs and books to help people take charge of their dog's and cat's health.

Our thanks and appreciation to Steve Brown, creator of Steve's Real Food and many other innovative products for dogs, for his work on analysis and food composition which helped us to give you these recipes.